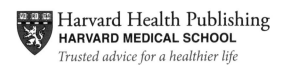

Harvard Health Publishing
HARVARD MEDICAL SCHOOL
Trusted advice for a healthier life

MW01046932

Dear Reader,

Among conditions that are both painful and non-life-threatening, back pain is one of the most common, affecting four out of five Americans at some point in their lives. And many of us—myself included—have to be wary of recurrences. But the good news is that back pain need not govern how you live your life.

Thanks to the pioneering work of back pain researchers, treatment has undergone a sea change. We now appreciate the central role of exercise in treating back problems and maintaining a healthy back. We also know that the best strategy to prevent repeat episodes of back pain is to reduce your risk factors—for example, by losing excess weight and becoming more physically active. This is good news both for people suffering with back pain and for society at large, because the overall costs of this common condition are staggering, with some estimates of lost wages and other economic costs exceeding $100 billion in the United States alone.

If you suffer from back pain, a program of medication, exercise, and lifestyle modification is likely to offer the most relief. Surgery is useful in select situations for patients whose conditions meet certain criteria. And if you are a candidate for surgery, you may find that you have options for minimally invasive procedures that can reduce surgical risk and have you on your feet and getting on with your life in just a few days.

This report describes common types of back problems and the treatments that are likely to relieve them. Our Special Section is devoted to self-help information on exercises, healthy back habits, and strategies like choosing the right mattress or chair. We also discuss the evidence for complementary therapies such as chiropractic care, acupuncture, and massage.

Most back pain isn't dangerous, but it's important to learn the "red flag" situations that require immediate medical attention. Once these have been ruled out, you and your health care team can choose the right treatment for your condition and your particular lifestyle. There are numerous options, but one thing is clear: your engagement in and determination to stick with a treatment program is vital, especially when it comes to exercise. So please work closely with your health care team as you evaluate the information in this report and find an approach that feels right for you.

Sincerely,

Jeffrey N. Katz, M.D., M.Sc.
Medical Editor

Harvard Health Publishing | Harvard Medical School | 4 Blackfan Circle, 4th Floor | Boston, MA 02115

Why is back pain so common?

At some time in their lives, most people will suffer back pain—usually in the lower back, also known as the lumbar region of the spine (see Figure 1, page 3). Low back pain is so common that when people speak of back pain, that's usually what they mean, although it's also possible to develop pain in the upper back (the thoracic spine) or the neck (the cervical spine). Because most cases are in the lower back, we will use the term "back pain" in this report to refer to low back pain, unless otherwise specified.

Though it's a common problem, back pain in general remains something of a medical puzzle. Even after extensive tests, physicians are often unable to pinpoint an exact cause. Many people with back pain visit one doctor after another, only to come away with conflicting opinions. All too often, the pain is ultimately classified as "idiopathic," meaning it has no known cause—yet it is all too real to the person affected.

Why is back pain such an enigma? It is important to understand that back pain does not describe a single entity. Instead, it is an umbrella term that includes a number of medical conditions that can vary in severity. In fact, some of these conditions don't even originate in the back, but are related to problems in other organs, such as the liver, kidneys, or aorta.

The way you manage your symptoms will depend on the type of condition you have and whether it is acute or chronic. Acute back pain comes on suddenly but usually gets better in a matter of weeks. If your back pain lasts more than three months with no improvement—or even gets worse—then the condition is considered chronic. Either way, one thing is clear: to regain your get-up-and-go, you need to do just that—get moving and stay physically active, within reason. And as is often the case in medicine, the more actively you participate in your treatment, the better your recovery is likely to be.

When back pain strikes, it's best to start with conservative treatments—unless certain "red flag" symp-

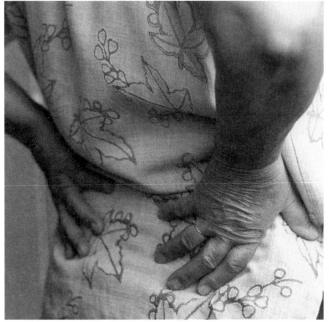

Back pain can develop for a variety of reasons. There are some risk factors that you can't change. However, a number of lifestyle changes either may lessen back pain or help you cope better.

toms suggest something more serious (see "'Red flag' symptoms and conditions," page 13). Conservative treatment usually means heat or ice and over-the-counter pain relievers as needed. If those don't work, there are other options, especially for people suffering chronic back pain. Though it's not always possible to eliminate the pain permanently, you can do a great deal to make flare-ups less painful and less frequent. This report will show you how.

What puts you at risk for back pain?

Although anyone can develop a backache, regardless of health or circumstances, research has found that some conditions or activities, known as risk factors, put you at greater risk for back problems. Some risk factors are things you can change; others you can't. But knowing the risk factors you can actually modify will allow you to take action to improve your back health.

Risk factors you can't change

No matter what you do, some risk factors for back pain are beyond your control, such as your age, your sex, and family history.

Age. Although back pain can affect people at any age, it's more common in midlife. This is when changes occur in the bones and joints of your back, even if you have never had a back injury. For one thing, the spinal discs—the structures that serve as cushions between the bones in the spine—tend to wear out and lose their ability to absorb the forces transmitted along the spine. These changes to the discs can cause pain.

Later in life, osteoporosis (loss of bone density)

Figure 1: Regions of the spine

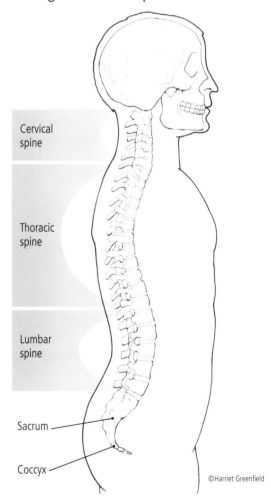

©Harriet Greenfield

Your spine is divided into three regions: the cervical, the thoracic, and the lumbar. Low back pain originates in the lumbar area, which extends from the bottom of your rib cage to your sacrum (the triangular bone at the rear of the pelvis). For more information, see "The anatomy of your back," page 6.

can become a problem. Osteoporosis can weaken the spinal bones (vertebrae) and make them more likely to break (fracture). In addition to being very painful, vertebral fractures can cause a loss of height and a rounding of the back.

While back pain problems are more common in people in their middle years, in older individuals back pain attacks are more severe and last longer. One reason is that older people are more likely to develop back conditions that are more serious and harder to treat than those common in middle age. One example is spinal stenosis, in which the spinal canal narrows and presses on nerves.

Sex. Studies suggest that back pain plagues men and women equally. However, the types of back pain they have may differ.

In Western industrialized societies, men are more apt to suffer from disc problems, and they are more likely to end up having surgery. These differences probably reflect the fact that more men than women work in jobs that involve heavy lifting, pushing, and pulling.

On the other hand, women often have backaches during pregnancy, particularly during the final trimester. And although the discomfort usually lessens and disappears after childbirth, it can become chronic. The exact reason for pregnancy-related back pain is unknown, but several factors probably contribute: ligaments normally loosen during the third trimester, abdominal muscles stretch and weaken, and carrying the developing baby and giving birth stress the back. Following childbirth, caring for an infant or small child further taxes the lower back.

A number of other back conditions are also more common in women. Because women have a higher prevalence of osteoporosis, they are more likely to have vertebral fractures. Women are also especially susceptible to degenerative arthritis of the lower spine, a condition that generally involves the vertebral joints. Finally, they are more likely to develop spondylolisthesis (see page 12), in which one vertebra slides forward relative to the one below it.

Family history. Heredity appears to play a role in certain types of back pain. Defects of the discs seem more common in some families. This may reflect a hereditary difference in the chemical makeup of discs that make them more prone to break down over time. Two other back conditions that tend to run in families are ankylosing spondylitis (see "Arthritis, including ankylosing spondylitis," page 12) and spondylolisthesis.

Risk factors you can change

Although you can't change your genes, sex, or age, you can change your lifestyle in ways that may lessen back pain or help you to cope with it better.

Work and play. Certain jobs and activities put a greater strain on your back. Work that involves long-term travel in motor vehicles is notoriously hard on the back, for instance, because it involves prolonged periods of sitting and exposure to vibration. The sitting positions necessary for office work—from typing to computer programming—can also eventually take a toll on your back regardless of your age.

Several other job-related activities increase the likelihood of future back problems:

- lifting or forceful movements such as pulling and pushing
- frequent bending or twisting of the back
- heavy physical exertion
- maintaining the same position for long periods
- repetitive motion patterns
- prolonged exposure to vibration.

Smoking. Smokers are at greater risk for back pain, possibly because smoking damages blood vessels that bring nutrients to the spine. Smokers are also much more likely than nonsmokers to develop chronic, disabling back pain.

Physical characteristics and posture. The good news is that your build, weight, and height seem to have little to do with your likelihood of developing back pain in the first place. Even a moderate difference in leg length—up to three-quarters of an inch—doesn't appear to make a difference. And despite your parents' admonition to "sit up straight," experts now agree that, in most cases, posture alone, whether bad or good, will neither predispose you to back pain nor shield you from it. Slumping and slouching don't seem to have much effect on the basic health of your spine.

But before you slump back in your chair, note that poor posture can worsen existing pain. Improving your body mechanics can help relieve your symptoms and prevent flare-ups (see "Building muscles," page 26, and

When studies conflict, what should you believe?

Hardly a day goes by without a headline in the health media about the results of a new study. Often the news is that what we thought was healthy (or unhealthy) actually isn't. Then, a year later, another headline comes along to say just the opposite. Who's right?

The results of studies do differ. Sometimes it's because of the way a study was designed. For example, studies of new drugs are more likely to show benefits if the drug is tested on people with severe cases of a disease rather than those with mild or moderate cases. The sicker people have more to gain, and therefore any small improvement over the usual treatment tends to stand out. Other times a study is just not very well designed or carried out, although this does not always stop the health press from seizing on a controversial finding and hyping it.

This Special Health Report attempts to reduce the confusion and mixed messages by relying whenever possible on two special kinds of scientific tools: meta-analyses and systematic reviews. These are "studies of studies" that pool findings from multiple previous pieces of research. The result is a kind of progress report on what scientists think they know about a health issue.

The prestigious Cochrane Collaboration is known for its systematic reviews, and its work is cited often in this report. It's a global network of health practitioners, researchers, patient advocates, and others who help to conduct comprehensive reviews of the scientific studies on a topic, both published and unpublished.

A meta-analysis gathers a smaller selection of studies than a systematic review, but it attempts to pool their findings into a result that is stronger than that of any individual one.

These tools help doctors and their patients make better decisions. They answer the question, "Based on the best studies conducted to date, does this particular treatment work—or does it work better than other existing treatments?" An individual study may say "yes" or "no," but systematic reviews and meta-analyses can sometimes demonstrate the old saying that there's strength in numbers.

"Stretching," page 26). Being physically out of condition is an important reason people have recurring bouts of the "sprain and strain" type of back pain (see "Sprains and strains," page 10).

And note that being overweight puts you at increased risk of having your symptoms return. What's the connection? Doctors aren't sure. Although it seems logical to think that carrying extra body weight causes back pain by increasing the strain on the spine, the connection may be more complicated than that. For example, becoming overweight tends to make you less physically active, and that could make back pain more likely.

Psychological factors. A growing body of evidence shows that emotions and psychological well-being have a significant influence on physical health. It is not surprising, therefore, to learn that these factors also affect the risk of having back problems. Psychological factors such as stress, anxiety, and negative mood and emotions all increase the likelihood of developing back pain.

For example, people who are unhappy at work because a job is unfulfilling or the pay is low tend to develop more back problems than the general population. The reasons for this are not completely understood. Part of the answer may lie in the fact that chronic pain and depression share some of the same biochemical roots. Imbalances in the neurotransmitters serotonin and norepinephrine, for example, play a role in mood disorders such as depression but also are involved in producing the sensation of pain.

fastfact | Not only is low back pain the most common cause of work-related disability for people under age 45, but it is also the most costly. Expenses to individuals include lost wages and medical bills, and companies shoulder expenses related to worker compensation.

Anxiety and depression can also sensitize people to pain, making them feel worse. Sleep deprivation can intensify the subjective perception of pain, too, so if sleep disturbances accompany the anxiety or depression, that would suggest another way in which psychological factors contribute to back pain. Psychological factors seem to be especially important in determining whether an acute bout of back pain will become a chronic problem.

Not surprisingly, the reverse is also true. Not only do people with psychological distress develop more back pain, but people with chronic back pain are three times more likely to be depressed and often suffer anxiety, stress, and sleep disturbances.

Fortunately, this dynamic can often be reversed with cognitive behavioral therapy (CBT; see "The mind-body connection," page 31). In CBT, a counselor helps you recognize negative thoughts, behaviors, and feelings and respond in a more positive way. Learning these coping skills can alleviate acute back pain and prevent it from becoming a long-term problem. People in the midst of a painful back pain flare-up, but who expect to improve over time, tend to do better. Moreover, a "can do" attitude can motivate you to start—and stick to—a program of stretching and strengthening exercises to ward off future episodes of back pain. Research on this intriguing topic continues, but remember that there is no known downside to being a happier person—regardless of its possible effects on your aching back. ◗

The anatomy of your back

To understand why back pain develops, it can help to know a little about the anatomy of the back. Vertebrae, discs, ligaments, muscles, and nerves form a complex structure that enables you to twist, turn, bend, stand, walk, run, and lift. But the back's complexity also makes it vulnerable. In particular, the lower part of the spine supports most of your body's weight and is subjected to great stress when you perform normal daily activities.

Vertebrae

The human spine consists primarily of a column of interlocking bones called vertebrae (derived from the Latin verb *vertere*, meaning "to turn"). Each vertebra is a roughly cylindrical body with a bony ring attached to its back surface. Spiky projections called processes extend in several directions from this ring. Vertebrae are stacked on top of each other, and ligaments link them together to form joints (see Figure 2, page 7). These joints permit a small amount of forward, backward, and side-to-side bending, as well as some twisting and up-and-down movement.

The lower, or lumbar, spine consists of the lowest five vertebrae (L1 through L5; see Figure 1, page 3). It extends from the bottom of the rib cage to the sacrum (the large triangular bone found between your hip bones) and connects your upper and lower body. Lumbago, a general term for low back pain caused by sprain or strain of unknown origin, affects the lumbar region of the back.

Discs: Your back's shock absorbers

A disc is tucked between each pair of vertebrae. These discs serve as small shock-absorbing cushions, help the spine to bend, and prevent the vertebrae from scraping against each other. Each disc has a gelatinous central part (the nucleus) and a tougher multilayered fibrous outer

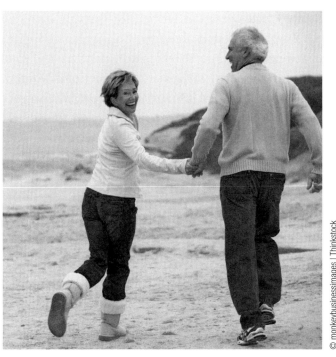

The back's complex design enables you to do twist, turn, run, walk, and lift. But that same complexity also makes your back vulnerable to a range of problems.

covering (the annulus) that binds to the adjacent vertebrae. The disc is fairly stiff over all, but pliant enough to absorb the forces exerted on the spine by daily life and protect the spinal column, with its precious spinal cord.

In view of the many stresses exerted on the lumbar spine throughout your life, it is little wonder that physical damage and age-related changes to the discs cause so many back problems. Indeed, the discs usually start to change after age 30. On the inside, the nucleus begins to dry out, harden, and lose its gelatinous consistency. On the outside, the annulus tends to fragment as its various layers break down. During the early stages of this process, the mechanical integrity of the disc gradually deteriorates, like a tire losing air. This reduces the disc's ability to absorb shocks, leaving the joint between the affected vertebrae more vulnerable to the physical forces exerted on it by everyday activities.

A flexible, protective column

Together, the vertebrae and discs form the spinal column. But what makes this stack of vertebrae and discs both strong and flexible? Ligaments connecting the vertebrae provide part of the answer. In addition, the rear portions of the vertebrae—the knobby parts you can feel under the skin on your back—interlock as well. These bony protrusions are called processes.

Multiple processes stick out from each vertebra. Each vertebra normally has seven: a spinous process at the middle of the back, two superior (upper) and two inferior (lower) articular processes, and right and left transverse processes on the sides (see Figure 2, below). The four articular processes mesh with those of adjacent vertebrae to form a series of small connections, called facet joints, which give the spine additional stability and also allow it to bend. The result is a strong but flexible tube of bone and ligament that extends from your head to your pelvis. It serves as a conduit that protects the spinal cord and permits the nerve roots to exit at the appropriate levels.

Muscles, ligaments, and tendons

Many muscles and ligaments connect to the bony processes of the vertebrae. The muscles apply the forces to your back that cause it to move, bend, twist, and stretch. They also limit and control back motions and support the spine—a bit like guy wires that support a tall television relay tower. This is why it's so important to exercise to keep the muscles that support and move the spine in good condition. The muscles that collectively support your spine can be divided into three general groups (see Figure 3, page 8).

Iliopsoas. These muscles, one pair on each side of the lumbar vertebrae, are attached to the vertebrae and to the inside of your pelvis. They pass downward in front of your hip joints and attach to the thighbones.

Figure 2: A closer look at your lumbar vertebrae

Side view

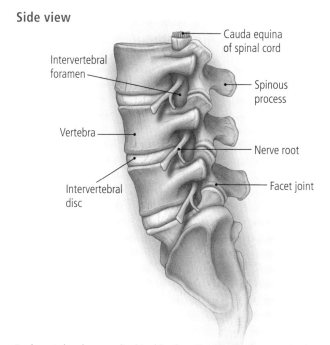

Each vertebra has a cylindrical body with a bony ring attached to its back surface as well as bony processes that project out in different directions from this ring. Intervertebral discs, tucked between each pair of vertebrae, serve as shock absorbers.

Cross-sectional view

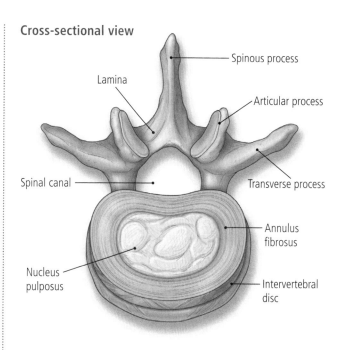

Each intervertebral disc has a gelatinous central part, called the nucleus pulposus, and a fibrous covering, called the annulus fibrosus. Each vertebra normally has seven spiky projections called processes that help stabilize your spine (five are shown above; the two lower articular processes are not visible in this illustration).

These muscles not only support your spine but also flex your hips and help balance your trunk on your lower limbs when you stand.

Erector spinae. These muscles (whose collective name comes from the Latin for "upholds the spine") are located to the left and right of your spine in the rear. They are the large muscle masses visible in the lower part of your back. The many different muscle groups of the erector spinae are anchored to the bony processes on the vertebrae, as well as to the pelvis below and the rib cage and thoracic and cervical spines above. They are the major supports of your spine during lifting.

During a sudden, new bout of acute back pain, these muscles may clench up tightly (spasm).

Abdominal muscles. Although these large muscles are not directly attached to the spine, they contribute a lot to the stability of the back. The flat abdominal muscles in front are attached to the pelvis below and the ribs above. These muscles form the cavity that contains your stomach and other abdominal organs. Since the abdominal muscles directly support the abdominal cavity, which is just in front of the spine, these muscles also provide indirect support to the lumbar spine.

Figure 3: Your back muscles and nerves

Supporting muscles

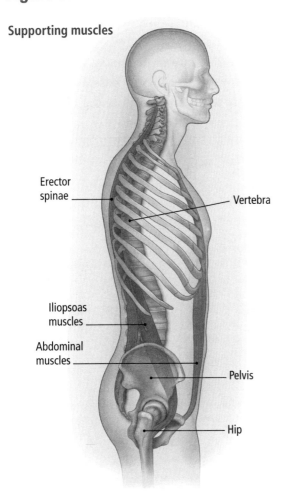

Nerves

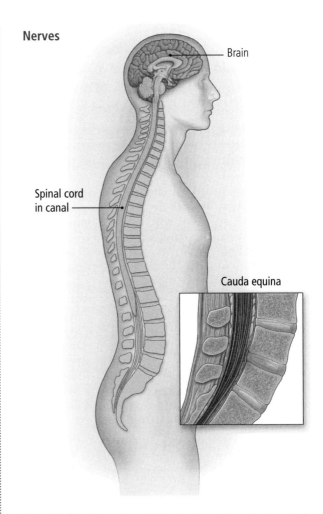

Three groups of muscles—the erector spinae, abdominal muscles, and iliopsoas muscles—support your spine and control back movements. The abdominal muscles span the abdominal cavity from the pelvis to the rib cage. The iliopsoas muscles allow you to flex your hips and help balance your trunk when you're standing.

The spinal cord runs from the brain down through the spinal canal and ends in the upper lumbar area. Nerve roots exit through the two narrow channels, one on each side, between adjacent vertebrae. In the lumbar spine, the lowermost nerve roots form a bundle of strands that resemble a horse's tail—in Latin, the *cauda equina*.

Each of these muscles connects to bone via tendons, and the many bones of the spine are anchored to one another with ligaments. Overuse and injury of these tendons and ligaments are common problems that likely account for many cases of back pain. Fortunately, such injuries generally heal over time (see "Sprains and strains," page 10).

Nerves

The spinal cord, or central nerve trunk, extends from the brain to the upper lumbar part of the spine. However, nerve roots continue downward to the end of the spine. The nerve roots in the lumbar spinal canal form a bundle of strands resembling a horse's tail and therefore are known by the name cauda equina, which is Latin for "horse's tail" (see the righthand illustration in Figure 3, page 8).

The cauda equina contains nerve fibers that control the leg muscles and play important roles in bladder, intestinal, and genital functions. Similarly, the sensory nerve fibers in the cauda equina provide feeling from some regions of the feet and legs as well as the bowel and bladder, enabling sensations to travel from the lower half of your body to your spinal cord and from there to your brain.

The vertebrae form the armored channel, or canal, that protects the nerve roots and spinal cord. However, certain problems in the vertebrae may endanger these very structures. For example, an opening can become too narrow, pressing on or pinching the nerve roots and their related nerve tissues. Compressed or irritated nerve roots within or near the lumbar vertebrae may cause low back or leg pain.

Various types of problems can cause this painful situation, known as nerve-root compression. For example, a bulging spinal disc can pinch a nerve or protrude into the spinal canal. Degenerative arthritis of the small joints in the spinal column, coupled with the formation of small bony growths (called osteophytes) around them, can also compress nerve roots. This problem is especially likely to occur in the two narrow channels, one on each side, between adjacent vertebrae, known as the intervertebral foramina. ♥

Types of back pain

Does this sound familiar? One day, you wake up and something feels different in your lower back—a twinge, a tightness, a warm ache. You try to gently stretch it out, but it's no use: by the end of the day you are hunched over in pain.

Why does your back hurt on this day but not another day? Although many episodes of back pain can be associated with a specific event—a fall, a sudden off-balance movement, or overdoing it in the garden or at work—it can be difficult to trace new back pain to a specific anatomical cause.

Even so, your doctor can often accurately diagnose a particular back pain condition and suggest appropriate treatments based on the type and the location of the pain (see "Diagnosing back pain," page 16). When the treatment is appropriate for the problem, recovery should go smoothly. With a mismatch, however, recovery may falter (see "Creating a treatment strategy," page 20).

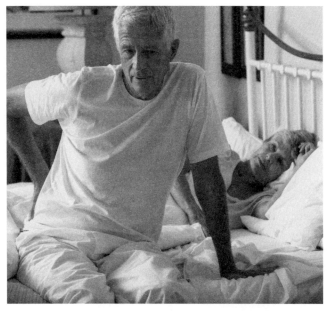

The most common causes of back pain are sprains (injuries to the ligaments in your back) and strains (injuries to the muscles or tendons). Sometimes you can relieve the comfort by lying down, but it's best to keep physically active.

Following is some basic information on the major types of back pain.

Sprains and strains

Sprains and strains are the most frequent causes of backaches. Sprains affect ligaments, the tough, fibrous bands of tissue found where bones, such as the vertebrae in your spine, connect at joints. Strains are injuries of either your muscles or tendons (which connect muscles to bones).

If you have a sprain or strain, the typical symptoms are tightness, stiffness, and painful muscle contractions, known as spasms. Because you may find it hurts to move, you are likely to limit your movements or to be more guarded when making them. Sometimes the only way to relieve this discomfort is by lying down—or sitting up straight, or standing. It varies from person to person and from one injury to the next.

Though sprains and strains are common, it is not always easy to diagnose them quickly and accurately. Your doctor will look for certain telltale symptoms: a "bent over" forward or sideways posture, limitations on how much you can move, and spasms in your chest and back muscles. Usually, there is no clear evidence of an irritated or compressed nerve—such as muscle weakness, diminished reflexes, or numbness and tingling. Medical imaging techniques, such as x-rays or MRI scans, are not useful for diagnosing strains and sprains. An x-ray, for example, won't show any abnormality or may show an abnormality that is unrelated to the symptoms.

▶ **Symptoms of back sprain or strain**

✔ Tightness

✔ Stiffness

✔ Muscle spasm

✔ Pain when moving your torso

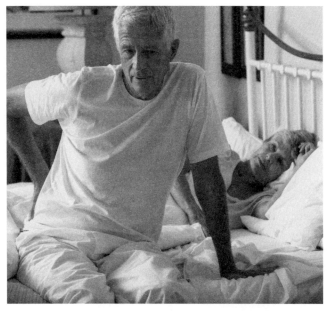

© Mark Bowden | Thinkstock

Nerve-compression syndromes

The next most common cause of back pain is a compressed or "pinched" nerve. Two common types of nerve-compression syndromes are disc problems (such as a herniated disc) and spinal stenosis, which occurs when a narrowing of the spinal column puts pressure on nerves in the spine.

Disc problems

Anyone at any age can injure one of the cushioning discs between the vertebrae, either through an accident or by pushing the discs beyond their limits during work or recreation. But over all, disc troubles become more common in middle age and beyond.

As a disc degenerates, the gelatinous center tends to lose water and become stiffer. In addition, a disc's outer shell (the annulus), which binds to the adjacent vertebrae, may weaken, become thinner, and begin to tear—especially in the parts of the disc closest to

Figure 4: Sciatica: Roots of the problem

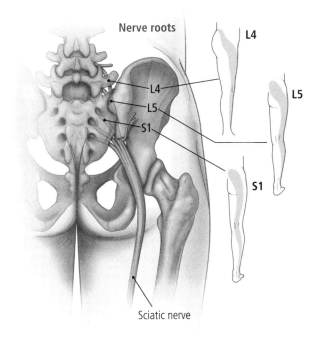

Nerve roots exit from between vertebrae in the spine. At the lower spine, five nerve roots merge to form the sciatic nerve in the leg. If a bulging disc pinches one of these nerve roots—especially lumbar 4 (L4), lumbar 5 (L5), or sacral 1 (S1)—it causes sciatica, sharp pain that typically radiates down the leg. You feel the pain in different areas, depending on which nerve root is pinched by the bulging disc.

► Symptoms of disc herniation

- ✔ Slight to intense pain in the back
- ✔ Shooting pain in the leg
- ✔ Possibly, numbness or weakness in the buttocks or legs

where the nerve roots exit the spinal column. A disc with these kinds of changes tends to bulge outward like an underinflated tire. Eventually, a portion of the inner disc material may protrude through a tear in the annulus, forming a herniation. People commonly refer to a herniated disc as a "slipped" or "ruptured" disc. The herniation may press on a nearby nerve root, leading to inflammation and back pain.

One characteristic form of pain from a herniated disc is called sciatica. This term refers to pain along the sciatic nerve, which passes through the buttock, down the leg, and into the foot (see Figure 4, at left). Sciatica may also include a sensation of pins and needles in the affected leg, especially in the foot and toes. A person with sciatica will typically assume a more rigid posture when sitting or standing to avoid pain.

The symptoms of a herniated disc vary. You may feel sharp pain when coughing or sneezing, or doing anything that pulls on the sciatic nerve, such as bending forward from your waist or flexing your hips while keeping your knees straight. If the pain is constant, it will be difficult to find a comfortable position. If the pain is occasional, sharp, and shooting, it will feel like an electric shock.

To confirm the diagnosis of a herniated disc and pinpoint the disc in question, your doctor will carefully assess your symptoms. In addition, diagnostic imaging (usually MRI scanning, but sometimes CT scanning) is often used. However, this practice, although still quite common, has come under scrutiny by health care quality experts. Many people walk around with discs that look abnormal in medical scans and yet experience no pain or other symptoms. In fact, if you were to scan the backs of all adults, one in four would show some degree of disc herniation. All that means is that the discs are aging. And the disc that looks most abnormal on an imaging scan might not be the one causing the

Symptoms of spinal stenosis

✔ Pain in the lower back when standing up straight, bending backward, or walking

✔ Pain that subsides when sitting or bending forward

✔ Pain in the buttocks or legs

pain. You don't want to rush into treatments until you are sure what's causing the problem.

However, if acute sciatic pain persists without any improvement for more than one month, despite treatment, it may indicate the need for further evaluation and a different treatment approach.

Spinal stenosis

Spinal stenosis is a narrowing of the spinal canal, the channel in the vertebrae that the spinal cord passes through. As the space becomes more constricted, it compresses the nerves, causing pain and certain other characteristic symptoms. Spinal stenosis is more common in people over age 50, since age-related degenerative changes are often the source of the problem. However, some people who naturally have smaller spinal canals are more likely to develop the condition and to be diagnosed earlier in life.

Various factors can contribute to spinal canal narrowing. These include bulging discs, thickening of the ligaments that connect the vertebrae, or the protrusion of small bony growths known as osteophytes (commonly called bone spurs) into the spinal canal. Other possible causes include a displaced ligament, thickening of a vertebra's bony plate (the lamina), or Paget's disease (abnormal bone metabolism).

Lumbar spinal stenosis causes low back pain and usually discomfort in the thighs or lower legs when you stand up straight, bend backward, or walk even short distances—as little as 50 to 100 yards. It's common for people with stenosis to be more comfortable

Symptoms of ankylosing spondylitis

✔ Back pain and stiffness

✔ Over time, limited movement of the spine

when leaning forward (for example, when pushing a grocery cart or sitting).

Your doctor is usually able to diagnose spinal stenosis based on your symptoms, medical history, and physical exam. However, x-rays, an MRI scan, or a CT scan may help in assessing this condition.

Arthritis, including ankylosing spondylitis

Degenerative arthritis of the facet joints occurs most frequently in older people. It often causes varying degrees of back pain, usually intermittent, over months or years.

Another form of arthritis that causes back trouble is called ankylosing spondylitis (from the Greek *ankylos* for "bent," and *spondylos* for "vertebra"). It is characterized by inflammatory changes in the tissues of the spine, including the spinal ligaments and the vertebrae and other bones of the spine. In this painful and disabling condition, the spine becomes inflamed and stiff. It is especially bothersome in the morning and after inactivity.

Ankylosing spondylitis usually develops before age 40 and can be mistaken for a back strain or a disc problem when mild. Sometimes, people with this condition have pain in both sides of the lower back or pelvis. When severe, it can lead to increasing pain over time and eventually cause the bones of the spine to fuse together in a rigid structure. These areas are no longer able to bend or rotate, making the back stiff and rigid.

Spondylolisthesis

An anatomical defect can cause the front portion of a vertebra as well as the vertebra above it to slip forward out of normal alignment. The defect may be some-

Symptoms of spondylolisthesis

✔ Lower back pain

✔ Muscle tightness (particularly at the back of the thigh)

✔ Stiffness

✔ Pain in the thighs and buttocks

✔ Shooting pain down one or both legs

When to call your doctor

Call your doctor immediately if you have any "red flag" symptoms along with your back pain, such as

- fever
- sudden or worsening leg weakness
- bowel or bladder control problems
- numbness in your groin or anal area.

Call your doctor within a few days if

- your back pain is intense enough to prevent you from doing ordinary daily tasks, and it has lasted for more than three or four days.

Try home treatment if

- your back pain has lasted for less than three or four days and has not involved any of the "red flag" symptoms listed above.

▶ Symptoms of cauda equina syndrome

- ✔ Low back pain
- ✔ Pain in one or both legs
- ✔ Bowel or bladder incontinence (leaking)
- ✔ Numbness in the anal and genital area (saddle anesthesia)
- ✔ Impotence

thing you were born with or may result from an injury or degenerative changes over time, such as spinal stenosis. The misalignment, known as spondylolisthesis, can cause severe low back pain, as well as discomfort in the thighs and hips. You may also experience sciatica, usually in both legs.

Certain types of athletes—including weight lifters, football players, gymnasts, and sumo wrestlers—are especially prone to this ailment as a result of injuries. By contrast, anyone can develop degenerative spondylolisthesis, which is caused by deformation or yielding of the bone of the facet joints. This condition occurs because of gradual wear and tear of the discs, facet joints, and other structures, rather than heavy lifting or bending or straightening the joints in the back.

"Red flag" symptoms and conditions

Although a backache can come on suddenly and with a painful fury, it usually does not require a visit to the emergency room (see "When to call your doctor," above). However, sometimes back pain does call for immediate medical attention because it arises from an infection, cancer, or another serious problem. The following situations are "red flags" that indicate that you should see a doctor as soon as possible:

- leg weakness that comes on abruptly or gets progressively worse

- back pain that occurs at the same time as a fever
- loss of bowel or bladder control
- numbness in your groin or anal area
- inability to find a comfortable position for sitting or sleeping during times when you feel back pain
- pain that worsens instead of getting better.

It's especially important to see a doctor immediately if you have worsening weakness in the legs, a problem with bladder or bowel control, or numbness in the groin or anal area. These symptoms are typical of nerve irritation that could lead to irreversible damage if left untreated.

The conditions listed below are causes of "red flag" back pain. They are much less common than simple sprain-and-strain backaches or disc-related conditions, but they have more serious health consequences.

Cauda equina syndrome

On rare occasions, when disc herniation is severe and compresses several nerves at the same time, it may affect your bladder and bowel function, causing such symptoms as bowel incontinence and difficulty initiating a stream of urine. The nerve compression may also cause severe weakness in one or both legs. If you have these symptoms, see a doctor immediately to avoid possible serious nerve damage. You may need emergency surgery.

Vertebral fracture

A sudden fall or impact can fracture one or more vertebrae. Vertebral fracture is not simple to diagnose, but it's often associated with certain symptoms. The pain tends to be quite severe and disabling, and is usually localized to the area of the injured vertebra (rather than being diffuse and radiating). Seek help quickly if you suspect you have suffered a vertebral fracture, especially if you have numbness, urinary or bowel incontinence,

▶ Symptoms of vertebral fracture

- ✔ Upper or lower back pain, depending on the location of the fracture
- ✔ Pain that radiates to other areas
- ✔ Numbness or tingling
- ✔ Pain that increases with movement
- ✔ In rare cases, impaired bladder or bowel function

or weakness, since these problems suggest that a bone fragment is damaging the spinal cord or a nerve root. Treatment depends on the location and nature of the fracture. If a doctor determines that the fracture does not affect the spinal cord, a wait-and-watch approach is best in most cases. However, if the fracture leads to spinal compression, you may need surgery.

Osteoporotic fractures. In older people, especially women past menopause, bones may become weaker, more porous, and susceptible to breaks. If you have osteoporosis, one or more vertebrae may fracture even if no actual injury has occurred. When the bone is weakened enough, something as innocuous as lifting a gallon of milk or sneezing can trigger such a fracture. This type of injury is also referred to as a compression fracture because the broken vertebra may collapse under pressure, causing the spine to shorten.

fastfact | An estimated one in four postmenopausal American women has experienced a spinal fracture from osteoporosis.

When a compression fracture occurs, the back pain comes on suddenly and is sometimes severe and disabling. The discomfort tends to center on the fractured vertebra, but it may radiate around one or both sides of the torso. While movement increases pain, lying down typically relieves it.

Each year, osteoporosis causes more than half a million vertebral fractures. As many as two-thirds of these fractures go undiagnosed, often because people mistakenly attribute the pain to sprains or strains. Spinal fractures can result in a loss of height, a rounding of the back, and even labored breathing. Sometimes wearing a back brace can help ease the pain.

Infection

A rare cause of back pain is a bacterial infection in a disc (discitis), in the bone of one or more vertebrae (osteomyelitis), or in the facet joints (infectious arthritis). Bacteria can invade the spine from various sites via the bloodstream. The source might be a boil or another skin infection, a urinary tract infection, an abscessed tooth, or an unsterilized hypodermic needle. You're more likely to develop a spinal infection if your resistance is compromised by a condition such as liver failure, diabetes, or AIDS, or by medications that interfere with your immune system, such as steroids or anticancer drugs.

Back pain caused by a spinal infection is often severe, and its symptoms may include back muscle spasms, fever, and tenderness around the infected vertebrae.

Spinal tumor

Spinal cancer is rare, affecting fewer than one in 1,000 people with back pain. But when tumors grow in the back—whether they are cancerous (malignant) or not (benign)—they can be quite painful. Most spinal tumors develop after the spread (metastasis) of cancer that originated elsewhere, especially in the breast, lung, or prostate gland. Less often, tumors originate in the tissues of the spine (including bones and ligaments), while others start in the spinal cord or nerve roots.

Depending on its location, a spinal tumor may mimic, at least for a time, almost any other cause of back pain, including a strain or sprain, a disc problem, or a fracture. However, the discomfort caused by a tumor is often unrelenting, and it typically increases in intensity over time. Bed rest and the other measures that give at least temporary or partial relief to people with the common forms of backache tend not to be helpful for tumor pain.

▶ Symptoms of spinal infection

- ✔ Severe back pain
- ✔ Pain that radiates to other areas
- ✔ Fever and sweating
- ✔ Pain that increases with movement

Symptoms of a spinal tumor

✔ Back pain that grows worse over time

✔ Abnormal sensations of pain, numbness, or cold in the leg or ankle

Because such tumors are relatively rare and their symptoms can be so similar to those of other back ailments, the correct diagnosis is sometimes delayed.

Back pain from abdominal disorders

Some back pain originates outside the spine or related structures, but is felt there, much as a heart attack can cause pain in the left arm. This is called referred pain. Ordinarily, this type of pain comes and goes independent of motions or activities that put stress on the spine. Moreover, x-rays and other diagnostic tests show nothing that implicates the spine.

One particularly dangerous example of referred back pain is abdominal aortic aneurysm (AAA). This condition develops in the abdominal portion of the aorta, the large blood vessel that carries blood from your heart to your lower trunk and legs. A bulge (aneurysm) gradually forms in the weakened wall of the aorta. When the aneurysm grows large enough, it can cause pain in the back, belly, or side. Without immediate medical attention, the aneurysm can burst and lead to death. Risk factors for this condition include smoking, high blood pressure (hypertension), atherosclerosis, and a family history of the problem. AAA is five times more common in men than women and occurs most often in people over 60. If you are a man in your 60s, ask your doctor if you can benefit from having a one-time ultrasound screening test for AAA.

Disorders of various abdominal or pelvic organs, including the pancreas, kidneys, liver, or uterus, can also cause back pain. ♥

Diagnosing back pain

Most people experience back pain at some point in their lives, whether the cause is a muscle strain, a fall, heavy lifting, or a "pinched" nerve. When back pain strikes, consult a doctor *immediately* if you experience any "red flag" symptoms that could indicate a more serious medical problem (see "'Red flag' symptoms and conditions," page 13).

Otherwise, the best approach is usually to wait and see if the problem resolves on its own. If the pain does not improve after trying home remedies for a week or two, then talking to a doctor could be helpful. To learn what you can do to treat or prevent back pain, see the Special Section, "Beyond drugs and surgery—other ways to help your back," page 24.

If you decide to see a doctor about your back pain, your first stop is likely to be with your primary care physician. If your problem is already chronic or the symptoms indicate the need for a specialist's attention, your doctor might refer you to an orthopedist, rheumatologist, neurologist, or physiatrist. Physician assistants (PAs) and nurse practitioners (NPs) are also playing an increasingly prominent role in back care (see "It takes a team," page 21).

Your medical history and exam

Despite impressive diagnostic methods developed since the 1980s, the key to successful diagnosis of back problems remains seeing a physician who will take a detailed medical history and conduct a thorough examination.

A medical history includes a precise account of your back pain, such as its duration and intensity, whether it radiates down the legs, whether it is accompanied by numbness or tingling, whether it is worsened by coughing or sneezing, and whether it has occurred in the past.

The clinician will check for "red flag" symptoms and other signs that could indicate that you have an underlying infection or spinal tumor. Telltale clues include weight loss, fever, anemia, or a personal history of cancer or weakened immune system. Since nicotine is toxic to the spinal discs, your doctor may ask if you smoke. And because genes play a role in some types of back pain, your physician will want to know if you have a family history of back pain.

As part of the physical examination, your doctor will check the contour and range of motion of your back. He or she will also check your knee and ankle reflexes, look for weakness in certain muscles (particularly those in the legs), and check the sensation in your legs and feet.

To check for signs of irritation to the nerve roots of your spine, the doctor will gently raise your leg as you hold it straight. This motion tugs on the sciatic nerve, producing pain in your leg if the nerve root is inflamed or if a disc presses on it. The doctor can often figure out which nerve root or roots are affected based on the location of numbness and tingling (see Figure 4, page 11).

Diagnostic imaging: When it is and isn't useful

Although it's often tempting to enlist technology to identify the cause of back pain, the current scientific consensus is that diagnostic imaging is overused at the time symptoms first appear and not helpful for diagnosing garden-variety back pain. As a result, experts estimate, one-quarter of diagnostic imaging scans in people with short-term (acute) low back pain don't lead to any real benefit, like reduced pain or better day-to-day functioning.

The reason x-rays and CT or MRI scans are often unhelpful in diagnosing back pain is that they frequently find abnormalities that are unrelated to your back symptoms. For example, nearly two-thirds of MRI examinations of people with no back pain reveal disc bulges or protrusions in the lumbar spine. Similarly, in people over age 50, up to 90% of x-rays and other imaging scans will show aging-related abnormalities—like arthritis—that frequently are unrelated to the person's pain or discomfort.

In short, the scans often reveal signs of wear and tear in the spine that may not be the source of your pain. Such "just in case" medical imaging isn't free, and it has potential harms. It can waste time and even lead to additional unnecessary testing and, ultimately, unneeded treatments—including back surgery, which comes with serious risks. What's more, CT and MRI are expensive tests, a factor that becomes something to consider if you have a copayment or deductible requirement on your insurance plan. And in the end, it can serve little purpose, given that roughly 90% of people with back pain recover on their own without these expensive tests, often in a matter of weeks.

To avoid having unnecessary scans, be a savvy consumer. Studies suggest that doctors who own a stake in diagnostic imaging centers tend to order more imaging tests than doctors who refer their patients to centers owned by someone else. A good back doctor will not rush into unnecessary imaging, even though the demand for the imaging often comes from patients themselves.

The bottom line? Unless a physician suspects you have a health condition that needs immediate attention, it's wise to wait four to six weeks before considering sophisticated imaging tests. Chances are you'll recover on your own.

What tests can help diagnose back pain?

There are times when imaging tests are appropriate. If the pain becomes chronic—that is, it persists with little or no improvement for three months or more—imaging studies and other tests can help identify the source of the pain and rule out serious problems. If your doctor thinks you might have a serious condition such as a tumor, infection, or cauda equina syndrome, advanced medical imaging could save your life.

If you and your physician agree an imaging test may be helpful, here are some of the standard options.

X-rays

X-rays produce images of bones and of other parts of the body that are rich in calcium (see Figure 5, at left). Although x-rays provide information about the condition of the bony vertebrae, x-rays of the spine provide limited information about the discs, ligaments, muscles, and other soft tissues. Nonetheless, x-rays are indispensable for identifying fractures as well as changes in the bones associated with tumors, infections, and certain forms of arthritis. X-rays expose you to some radiation, but the doses are low. In the absence of other significant radiation exposure, occasional x-rays don't pose a significant danger.

Computed tomography (CT)

CT imaging provides distinct outlines of the various structures of the back (see Figure 6, page 18), such as the vertebrae. While CT scans can show arthritis or spinal narrowing (stenosis), they may not indicate clearly whether a herniated disc is causing a problem, such as sciatica.

Figure 5: X-ray of the spine

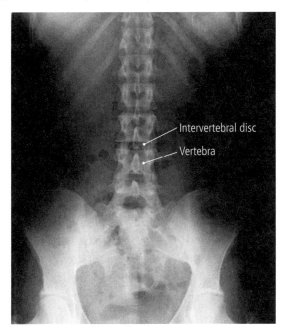

Intervertebral disc
Vertebra

An x-ray primarily shows bones and other tissues that contain calcium. While a single diagnostic x-ray exposes a person to a negligible amount of radiation, the exposure from a CT scan can be significantly higher.

Figure 6: CT scan

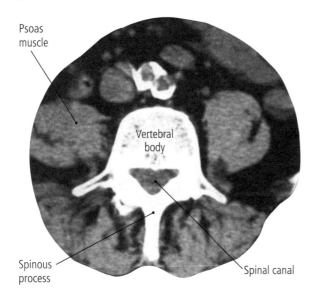

Psoas muscle

Vertebral body

Spinous process

Spinal canal

Computed tomography (CT) provides images of the body in different planes and shows distinct outlines of the various structures. A CT scan of the lumbar spine takes 10 to 15 minutes. The radiation exposure varies according to the type of equipment used and the size of the person being scanned.

CT scan courtesy of Daniel I. Rosenthal, M.D., Radiology Department, Massachusetts General Hospital.

During a CT scan, you must lie still for 10 to 15 minutes on a table that slides into a tunnel-like scanner. An x-ray device moves along your body taking multiple pictures from slightly different angles. Instead of sending a single x-ray beam through your body, this device uses many narrow beams. A detector that rotates around you collects the beams and sends the information to a specialized computer, which instantaneously analyzes and synthesizes multiple images of your back. The result is a set of remarkably detailed views. CT has one important downside: the scanning exposes you to much more radiation than a conventional x-ray.

Magnetic resonance imaging (MRI)

MRI technology uses electromagnetic waves to create images of your tissues, thus avoiding the radiation hazard of x-rays and CT scans. Unlike CT, MRI creates images of soft tissues, including intervertebral discs, spinal nerves, and tumors (see Figure 7, page 19).

The MRI procedure usually takes about 45 min-utes. You lie motionless on a table that slides into the center of the donut-shaped scanning machine. The machine bathes you in a strong magnetic field and probes the body's water-rich soft tissues with radio waves. The resulting scans are extremely detailed.

While in the MRI scanner "tunnel," you may feel anxious or claustrophobic. The machine makes unpleasantly loud buzzing, clicking, and knocking sounds, so you will wear ear protection. Diagnosing certain back problems may require an injection into your bloodstream of a special contrast dye before the scan. A small percentage of people have an allergic reaction to the dye. Unless you need to have the dye injected, MRI scans are not invasive and are believed to be harmless.

MRI scans are expensive, but when used in conjunction with a medical history and physical examination, MRI can eliminate some of the guesswork involved in making a diagnosis.

Myelography

Myelography is a form of diagnostic imaging that shows the positions of the lumbar nerve roots—the nerves that exit the spinal cord between pairs of vertebrae in the lower back. This sensitive procedure can also indicate distortions in the shape of the fluid-filled sheath that surrounds the spinal cord and the cauda equina.

It works this way: The doctor first injects a contrast medium (a fluid opaque to x-rays) into the spinal canal. This allows a type of x-ray machine called a fluoroscope to observe the flow of the contrast medium through the space around the cord and the nerve roots. The resulting images reveal abnormalities such as herniated discs, stenosis, or spinal tumors.

However, myelography is expensive and also invasive, since it requires puncturing the protective sheath around the spinal cord with a needle. Some people find it to be quite uncomfortable. Possible complications include headache (occasionally severe), an allergic reaction to the contrast fluid, and even infection resulting from the lumbar puncture, although this is rare. Myelography is performed only when a diagnosis is particularly difficult or when it's necessary to pinpoint the location of a problem in preparation for a complex surgery. In such cases, myelography can be done in combination with CT imaging.

Tests used less commonly to diagnose back pain

On occasion, a physician will recommend a bone scan or nerve conduction test. As with the tests already described, these are useful once your doctor has ruled out some probable causes of your pain and is therefore using the tests to further narrow the possibilities.

Bone scan. For this test, the doctor injects a short-lived radioactive substance called a tracer into your bloodstream. Your bones absorb this substance at rates that vary according to the level of biological activity in the bone cells. A tumor, an infection, or a healing fracture will appear as a "hot spot" on the bone scan image. Pinpointing the location of an abnormality makes it possible to use other techniques to provide a more definite diagnosis.

Bone scans take about four hours, starting from the time the tracer is injected. The exposure to radioactivity associated with this procedure is a fraction of that required for a regular x-ray of the lower spine. The only discomfort is in having the injection and lying facedown for up to an hour during the scan.

Electromyography and nerve conduction tests. For electromyography, fine needles are inserted into your muscles to detect and record electrical activity. This allows the doctor to diagnose pressure and irritation affecting the spinal nerves as well as certain diseases that can change the nature and speed of the signals. Electromyography requires multiple needle sticks

Figure 7: MRI scan

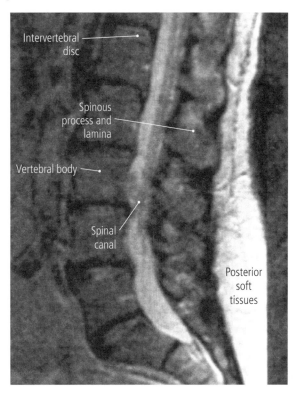

Intervertebral disc

Spinous process and lamina

Vertebral body

Spinal canal

Posterior soft tissues

Like CT, magnetic resonance imaging (MRI) provides images of your body in different planes. Unlike CT, it also shows soft tissues in some detail. An MRI scan of the spine takes about 45 minutes and does not involve any exposure to radiation.

MRI scan courtesy of Daniel I. Rosenthal, M.D., Radiology Department, Massachusetts General Hospital.

into the muscles, so it causes moderate discomfort.

Electromyography is often done along with nerve conduction testing, which determines how fast individual nerves relay signals. Together, electromyography and nerve conduction testing provide a more complete picture of the function of spinal nerve roots. ▼

Creating a treatment strategy

A wide variety of options exist for managing back pain. For new back pain or a flare-up of an existing "bad back," the most conservative strategy is to wait for the pain to resolve on its own while using conservative treatments like exercise, pain relievers, and heat or icing to soothe your discomfort. If the pain does not resolve, then your next step is to see a back pain specialist—usually an orthopedist—to obtain an accurate diagnosis of your problem.

At the most invasive end of the treatment spectrum, your doctor may recommend surgery for a painful, disabling, and chronic back problem that has failed to improve despite conservative treatment. For a discussion of treatment options, see the Special Section, "Beyond drugs and surgery—other ways to help your back," page 24; "Medications for back pain," page 36; and "When is surgery an option?" on page 42.

The scientific evidence for different treatments is not always cut-and-dried, but there are things you can do to get the best results:

First, get the most accurate diagnosis possible of the type of back disorder you suffer from (see "Types of back pain," page 10). An accurate diagnosis allows you to choose the treatment options appropriate for your specific problem—from conservative management to risky surgery.

Second, whether you're experiencing back pain for the first time or you've suffered a relapse, seek the advice of an experienced, certified, and well-recommended health specialist who understands your type of back problem. You could visit a primary care physician, orthopedist, rheumatologist, neurologist, neurosurgeon, or physiatrist (see "It takes a team," page 21).

Third, be an active participant in your care (see "What can you do?" on page 22). Shared decision making in health care means fully understanding the risks and benefits of the various treatments you are considering for your particular problem and any alternative treatments available.

Finally, don't be afraid to ask for a second opinion if your clinician recommends an invasive, experimental, or very expensive treatment. Doctors generally welcome your full participation in health care decisions and should support your request for a second opinion if you feel hesitant about a particular treatment.

Factors to consider

Ultimately the management strategy or treatment you choose to ease your back pain will depend on several variables. Chief among these are medical considerations, such as your back problem's likely course over time, whether the problem is short- or long-term, and your personal situation and preferences. Taking all these factors into account will help you and your clinician determine which of the available options are right for you.

Know your condition's timeline

Decades of medical practice and research have revealed much about the likely future course—or what doctors call the "natural history"—of various types of back pain. This includes how long a medical problem is likely to persist and how it will affect you if left untreated. This information is very helpful, especially if you're considering a surgical option. If painful flare-ups are likely to be brief and moderate, you might decide to hold off on surgery. If the natural history of your condition suggests that the timeline will be longer and more difficult, surgery might be an option worth more consideration.

In time, most backaches due to sprain or strain will get better without medical intervention, often within a week or two. Many people with nerve-compression problems will also benefit from a wait-and-watch approach. For example, 90% of people with sciatica or herniated discs will recover on their own within six months. By contrast, a condition like spi-

It takes a team

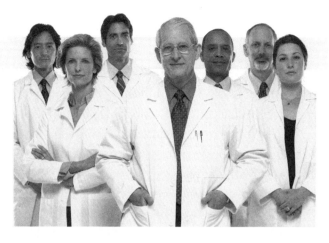

You may need to see more than one type of practitioner to alleviate back pain, starting with a generalist—often, a physician assistant or a nurse practitioner—and then seeking more specific types of help. Here's a quick guide to the types of clinicians you might encounter.

Generalists

Primary care physician: A medical doctor trained in general medicine, internal medicine, or family practice; makes referrals to specialists as necessary.

Physician assistant: A professional licensed by the state to diagnose and treat illness; works under the supervision of a physician in a physician's office, a hospital, or a clinic.

Nurse practitioner: A specially trained nurse licensed to diagnose and treat illness, often with a focus on prevention and wellness education.

Medical specialists and other practitioners

Chiropractor: A professional trained in manipulation of the bones and joints, including those in the spine.

Neurologist: A medical doctor who focuses on treatment of the nerves and nervous system.

Neurosurgeon: A medical doctor who provides surgical care for nerve-related problems.

Orthopedist: A medical doctor who diagnoses and treats problems of the skeletal system and its muscles, joints, and ligaments.

Osteopath: A doctor who has training similar to that of an M.D., but with an emphasis on the musculoskeletal system and the body's ability to heal itself.

Physiatrist: A medical doctor who specializes in rehabilitation.

Physical therapist: A professional who focuses on exercises and other rehabilitative techniques to restore function and mobility.

Rheumatologist: A medical doctor who specializes in the treatment of rheumatic diseases (those affecting the joints, muscles, bones, skin, and other tissues), some of which can affect the back.

---

nal stenosis, if left untreated, is less likely to improve over time and could get worse. Simply knowing the natural history of your condition will enable you to understand what is coming and make informed decisions about treating your pain.

Acute or chronic?

The likelihood that a back problem will improve on its own depends to a large extent on whether it's acute or chronic.

Acute back pain comes on suddenly. It may be triggered by something you did at work or at play. It can also be caused by a compressed nerve or a degenerative condition such as arthritis. Studies suggest that one-third of people with acute back pain from a sprain or strain will be much improved in as little as one week after the start of their symptoms. More often, however, painful backs mend more slowly, over four to eight weeks. Two-thirds of people will experience improvement within seven weeks.

Unfortunately, the problem often recurs: about 40% of people who develop low back pain will experience another bout of symptoms within six months. Therefore, after the initial acute episode resolves, prevention is key. (See the Special Section, page 24, for recommendations on back care.)

Chronic back pain by definition shows little or no improvement after three months. Often the precise cause of the pain is difficult to pinpoint, and it gets progressively worse. In general, chronic back pain responds best to a management plan that includes several different approaches—for example, a combination of pain-relieving medication, physical activity, and a complementary therapy such as acupuncture, massage, or yoga. You may need to visit a pain clinic in order to manage the pain. Work with your doctor to find the best combination for you. Your goal is to control pain and remain as functional as possible, so you can continue to live the life you want.

What can you do?

To be an active participant in your care, learn everything you can about your condition. Then help your doctor decide on a course of action that's best suited to you. Ideally, this "patient-centered care" means your expectations and preferences—not your doctor's—will guide your treatment plan.

Make your goals and preferences known to your doctor. How hard are you prepared to work at rehabilitation? Are you willing to do a lot of exercise? How reluctant are you to take medication? How anxious are you about surgery? What goals of treatment are the most important to you? Perhaps you can live without hiking in the mountains, but you still want to go on that long-awaited European trip.

Stick with treatment guidelines

Major medical societies periodically review the best available scientific data on how to treat conditions like back pain effectively. They then use that data to develop recommendations to guide clinicians. Although doctors naturally weigh treatment options on a case-by-case basis, expert guidelines help set standards for best practices.

For example, the American College of Radiology does not recommend immediate use of x-ray, CT, or MRI for assessing acute low back pain or sciatica. Also, the latest treatment guidelines from the American College of Physicians advise against prescribing narcotic prescription painkillers before trying acetaminophen (Tylenol) or nonsteroidal anti-inflammatory drugs (NSAIDs) like ibuprofen (Advil, Motrin) and naproxen (Aleve).

Yet research has spotted some contrary trends in back pain care: Doctors frequently order MRI, CT, and x-ray tests that, according to treatment guidelines, are unnecessary or are unlikely to ultimately help patients. More concerning, many people with acute low back pain are prescribed narcotic pain relievers prematurely.

The reasons why doctors don't always follow treatment guidelines are complex. Some of this so-called low-value care is driven by patients asking their doctors for "something stronger" than acetaminophen or NSAIDs, or insisting on an MRI or CT scan. But conservative care is worth a try before ramping up to more expensive and potentially risky options. To make informed decisions, ask your doctor to explain how likely a treatment is to help you—and how it could hurt you.

Look for a strategy that is suited to your situation. Just as there is no single cause of back pain, so too there is no one-size-fits-all solution. For example, your back pain may have been caused by an injury. In that case, you may choose to take pain-relieving medications as a first step, but then to work with a physical therapist to find ways to avoid a similar injury in the future. Or, your back pain may be related to a sedentary lifestyle; over time, your body has become deconditioned. If you are out of shape, you may start a regular walking routine to improve your overall physical condition. Perhaps you are having a hard time at work: low pay and job dissatisfaction influence back problems. In this case, it may be time to find ways to reduce your stress level or find a job that is more satisfying.

Whatever the case, your long-term strategy will depend on the condition itself and your preferences. You need to be very clear about what it is you want from treatment. These are some of the questions you could discuss with your doctor:

- Why do you think this is the best treatment for me?
- What are the risks of the treatment?
- What are the risks of not having the treatment right now?
- Are there more conservative options (if the recommended treatment is surgery)?

What can your doctor do?

Your doctor should provide appropriate and safe pain control. But you shouldn't expect or demand medications (such as narcotic painkillers) that your doctor says are inappropriate or risky (see "Stick with treatment guidelines," at left).

Your doctor should answer your questions and offer sufficient information about the risks and benefits of the various treatment options. Can he or she provide rough percentage estimates of how likely a treatment or surgery is to work? And how likely is it to go badly or lead to dangerous complications?

Your doctor can also provide referrals to other specialists who may help you (see "It takes a team," page 21). You can, for example, see a physical therapist for help with a chronic back condition. (Research suggests that physical therapy is not generally helpful for acute backaches but can be very useful for preventing recurrences or for treating chronic back pain.) A physical therapist can assess the nature and cause of musculoskeletal problems such as strain and sprain. The therapist can then suggest stretching and strengthening activities to address your particular problems. The aim is to strengthen abdominal and back muscles, preserve motion in the spine, reduce your pain, improve overall fitness, and prevent future problems. A variety of physical therapy approaches are available; ask your doctor for specific guidance and advice on what is most likely to help you.

If the pain persists, your doctor may refer you to a pain clinic. These centers use a variety of approaches, including education, cognitive behavioral therapy, exercise programs, biofeedback, relaxation techniques, and selective nerve blocks. These therapies can ease the pain or minimize its effect on your daily routine. The primary goal is to help you return to a more active life. ⬤

Beyond drugs and surgery—other ways to help your back

When it comes to deciding on an appropriate treatment approach for your back problem, you're in the driver's seat—with your doctor beside you as navigator. With all the options at your disposal, it's wise not to rush into a decision. If you allow yourself some time, your back problem may clear up in a few weeks or months with little or no medical intervention. Indeed, understanding how your condition is likely to progress over time is a critical precondition to making a good treatment decision.

But taking time to consider your options doesn't mean you do nothing. On the contrary, there's much you can do to ease your pain and speed your healing from the start, besides simply taking pain relievers. This chapter offers suggestions for effective self-care during an acute attack of back pain, along with complementary therapies you may wish to explore. To help prevent repeat episodes of back pain, it also includes various lifestyle strategies you can adopt.

First steps: Cold and heat

Applying moderate cold or heat to your back can reduce discomfort. It's best to use cold compresses or an ice pack, not heat, immediately following an injury. This numbs the pain somewhat and can prevent or reduce swelling (inflammation). About 48 hours after the onset of back pain, though, applying heat to your back may be more helpful. The warmth soothes and relaxes aching muscles. Heat also increases blood flow, which carries oxygen and nutrients to the

Extended bed rest is no longer recommended for sprains and strains. A limited amount of physical activity can actually help you recover faster.

© KatarzynaBialasiewicz | Thinkstock

injured area and thus promotes the healing process. Generally, electric heating pads and hot-water bottles are effective and easy to use. Heat therapy tends to help only in the early days of an acute attack (up to a week). Make sure not to apply heat or cold directly to exposed skin, and don't fall asleep while applying either one; skin damage may result.

Rest—but not too much

Extended bed rest was once a mainstay of treatment for low back pain, but no longer. Although lying in bed does minimize stress on the lumbar spine, extended bed rest creates other problems:

- Muscles lose conditioning and tone.
- Gastrointestinal problems, such as constipation, may arise.
- Blood clots may develop in the veins of the pelvis and legs, which raises the risk of pulmonary embolism (a serious medical condition in which a blood clot, usually dislodged from a vein in the pelvis or leg, blocks an artery in the lung).
- Depression and an increased sense of physical weakness and malaise may occur—a common phenomenon in people confined to bed rest.

For all these reasons, it's far better to engage in a limited amount of physical activity than to lie in bed. So get up regularly and walk around a bit, to the extent you can. Research shows that an early

return to work—with some restrictions or light duty, if necessary—is better for you than staying home from work for an extended period.

That said, some bed rest can be useful, particularly if you are in severe pain while sitting and standing. Try to restrict bed rest during the day to a few hours at a time, for no more than a couple of days. To ease the strain on your back, try putting pillows under your head and between your knees when lying on your side, under your knees when lying on your back, or under your hips when lying on your stomach. These positions reduce pressure on your back from sitting or standing—especially on the discs, ligaments, and muscles. Alternatively, you may be more comfortable sitting upright rather than lying down. Many people wonder whether a particular type

of mattress makes a difference, but there isn't much proof of this (see "Ask the doctor: What type of mattress is best for people with low back pain?" above).

Get moving

The sooner you can get up and moving, the faster you will recover. Exercise therapy can help the recovery process during an acute episode of back pain, prevent repeat backaches, and improve your day-to-day function even if you have chronic back pain.

Developing a suitable exercise program under expert supervision will enable you to build strong, flexible muscles that will be less prone to injury. If you have acute back pain, the goal is to help you resume normal activities as soon as possible and to remain symptom-free following recov-

ASK THE DOCTOR

Q *What type of mattress is best for people with low back pain?*

A Considering that most people spend roughly a third of their lives lying in bed, this is a very good question. In the past, doctors often recommended very firm mattresses. However, some studies have found that some people who sleep on hard mattresses have more back pain. On the other hand, while a softer mattress that conforms to your body's natural curves may help the joints align favorably, you might also sink in so deeply that your joints twist and become painful during the night. Something in the middle is often the best.

I usually advise my patients to try sleeping on different mattresses and beds to see if they can find a type that they like. If you spend a night at a hotel or someone else's house, make note of how you feel after sleeping on the "new" bed. You might also try placing a plywood board under your current mattress to dampen any movement from bedsprings, or put your mattress on the floor to simulate the feeling of a firm bed. Finally, go to a mattress showroom and try a variety of different models before buying a new one.

—*Jeffrey N. Katz, M.D.*

ery from the immediate attack. If you have chronic back pain, work with your physician to define your desired functional goal—whether it involves being able to tour museums, play with your grandchildren, or simply sit in the backyard reading a good book.

Any exercise program should be customized to meet your individual needs and introduced gradually a couple of weeks after the onset of symptoms or when you are feeling reasonably comfortable. One golden rule about any exercise program is to stop if it becomes painful. Exercise is meant to help, not hurt.

Another guiding principle of exercise for back pain is "start low and go slow." Begin with a low level of exercise that you can do without pain or strain and ramp up gradually. Walking is a good starter activity. Start with a duration you can easily tolerate, and then increase your time by 10% to 15% every week. Most people can double their walking time within five to six weeks.

If you were exercising before an episode of back pain and then had to slow down or stop for a while because of the pain, don't resume exercising at the same level as before the episode. If you try to pick up your exercise routine where you left off, you might injure yourself. Start by doing less (shorter duration or fewer repetitions) and gradually build back up to where you were before.

Building muscles

Aging and lack of exercise can leave you with weak, deconditioned back and abdominal muscles, triggering or worsening back pain. That's why stretching and strengthening these and other "core" muscles, which help to support the spine, is so important to recovering from back pain and preventing a recurrence of the problem.

A stretching and strengthening regimen should target the back, abdominal, buttock, and upper leg muscles (see "Back-strengthening exercises," page 27). Strong abdominal and back muscles, for example, help you maintain an upright posture and proper alignment of the spinal column. Meanwhile, the buttock muscles and the iliopsoas muscles (which run from the lumbar vertebrae to the hips on each side) help support the back during walking, standing, and sitting. In addition, the muscles of the upper legs should be strong and flexible, because they're connected to the iliopsoas and buttock muscles and, if weak and tight, can strain the supporting structures of the back.

Stretching

Stretching is a valuable component of any treatment plan for a person plagued by back problems. Most experts believe that supple, well-stretched muscles are less prone to injury. Indeed, shorter, less flexible muscle and connective tissues restrict joint mobility, which

increases the likelihood of sprains and strains.

Stretch regularly but gently, without bouncing, as that can cause tissue injury. Beginners should start by holding a stretch for a short time and gradually build up to roughly 30-second stretches.

What kind of stretch is best? Static stretching is when you stretch a muscle and hold for some period of time. Dynamic stretching is when you extend your limbs and move your joints through their range of motion—for example, doing "windmills" by rotating your outstretched arms. Despite continuing research, it remains unclear which type of stretch—static or dynamic—is best for back health in non-athletes. Some people like to warm up with dynamic stretches before exercising. Ask a physical therapist or sports medicine specialist for an individual recommendation.

Aerobic exercise and sports

In addition to doing exercises to make you stronger and more flexible in the lower back, you should also engage in regular aerobic exercise. This offers many benefits for general health and also helps prevent episodes of back pain.

Certain aerobic activities are safer for your back than others. Low-risk, high-benefit activities for most people's backs include bicycling (either stationary or moving), swimming, and walking. These low- or minimal-impact exercises

Back-strengthening exercises

The exercises below can help you reduce flare-ups of routine muscle-related back pain. These are standard exercises that are often used in physical therapy. Show this page to your back care provider and ask if these would be helpful for you. If so, perform each set of exercises every day after acute back pain subsides and your doctor says it's safe. Take it slow, and stop if it hurts.

Week 1: Getting started

Perform these exercises every day in the first week of your exercise program.

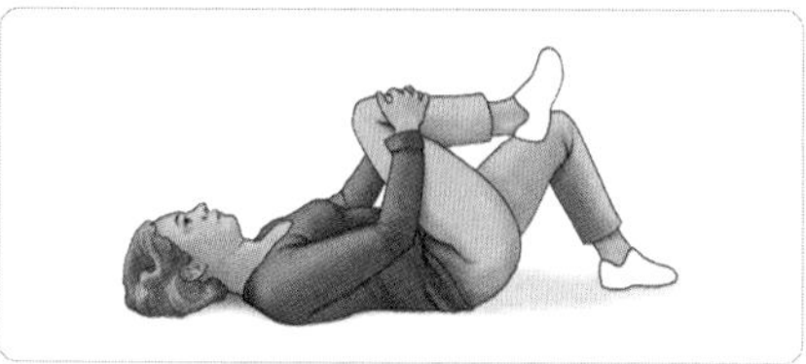

Lie on your back with both knees bent. Pull one knee toward your chest and hold it for 5 to 10 seconds. Return to the starting position. Repeat with the other leg. Do this 5 to 10 times with each leg.

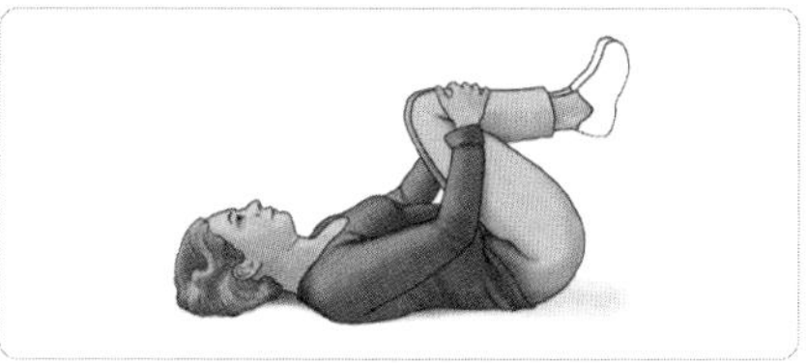

Lie on your back with both knees bent and your feet on the floor. Pull both knees toward your chest and hold for 5 to 10 seconds. Return to the starting position. Do this 5 to 10 times.

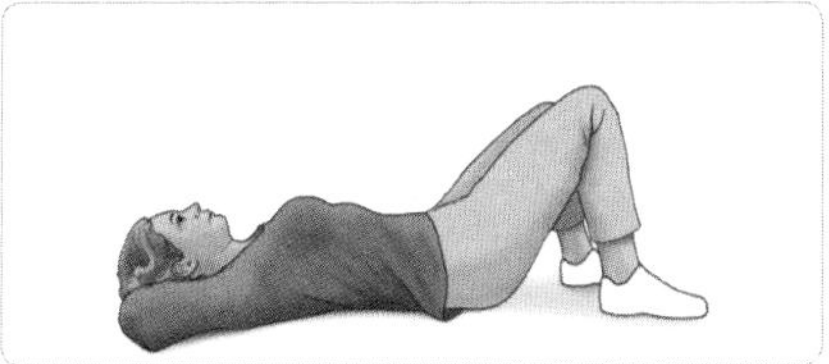

Lie on your back with both knees bent and your feet on the floor. Gently flatten your lower back to the floor and hold for 5 to 10 seconds, then relax. Do this 5 to 10 times.

Week 2: Taking it to the next level

If you do not feel any change in symptoms, such as worsening pain, add these three exercises every day starting the second week.

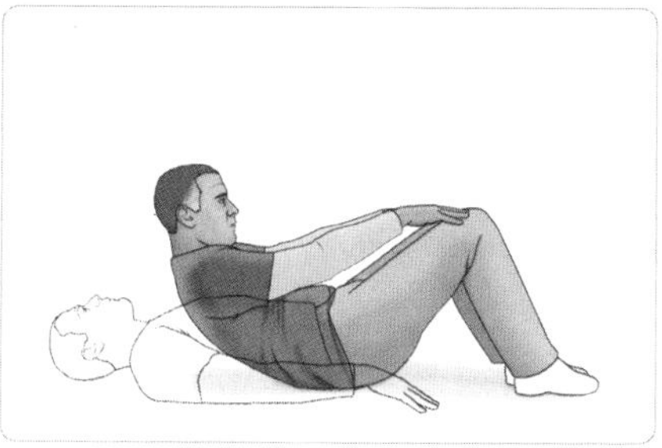

Lie on your back with both knees bent and your feet on the floor. Gently reach toward your knees, lifting your shoulders and head off the floor until your fingertips touch your knees. Hold this position for 5 to 10 seconds, then relax slowly back to the starting position. Do this 5 to 10 times.

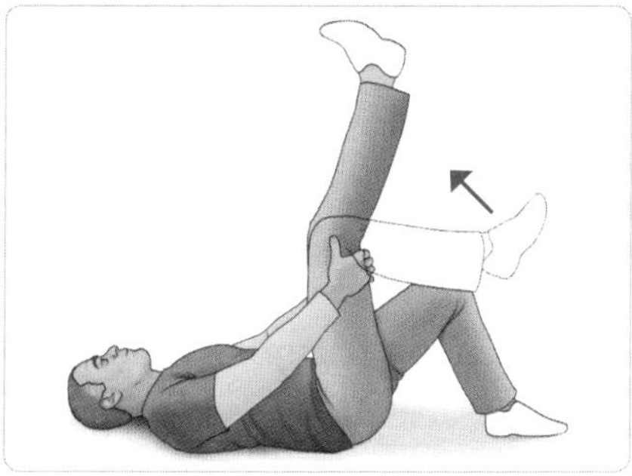

Lie on your back with both knees bent. Grasp the back of one leg behind the knee and pull it toward you, then very gently straighten the leg till it points vertically. Feel the stretch at the back of your thigh. Hold 5 to 10 seconds, then return to the starting position. Do this 5 to 10 times with each leg.

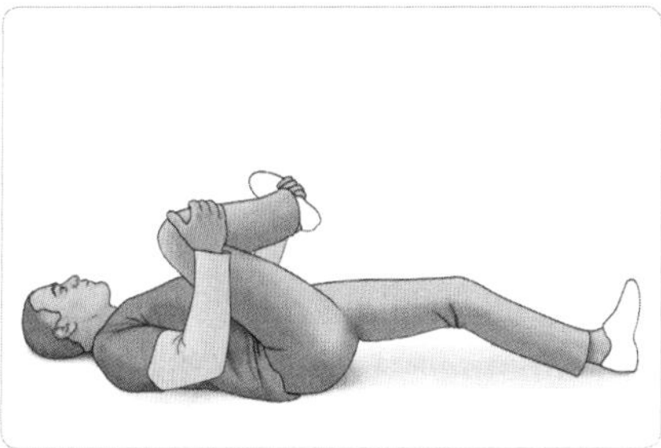

Lie on your back with your legs straight out. Bend your right knee and rotate your hip so that the lower leg is across your chest, pointing to the left. You should feel this stretch in your thigh. Hold for 5 to 10 seconds, then return to the starting position. Do this 5 times with each leg.

Week 3: Strengthening your core

If you are doing well on your new exercise regimen, add these core-strengthening moves in the third week.

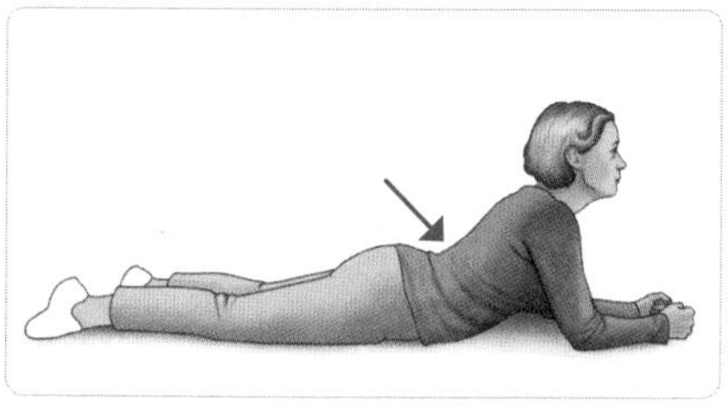

Lie face down on the floor, your bed, or an exercise mat. Bend your torso upward and rest the weight on your forearms. Gently arch your lower back and hold for 10 seconds, then relax. Repeat 5 to 10 times.

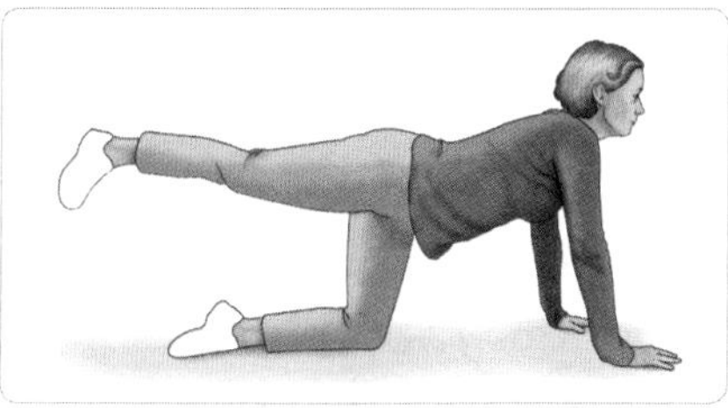

Start on your hands and knees. Lift and straighten one leg, extending it gently backward without lifting it above your body level. Hold the position for 5 seconds. Do this 5 to 10 times with each leg.

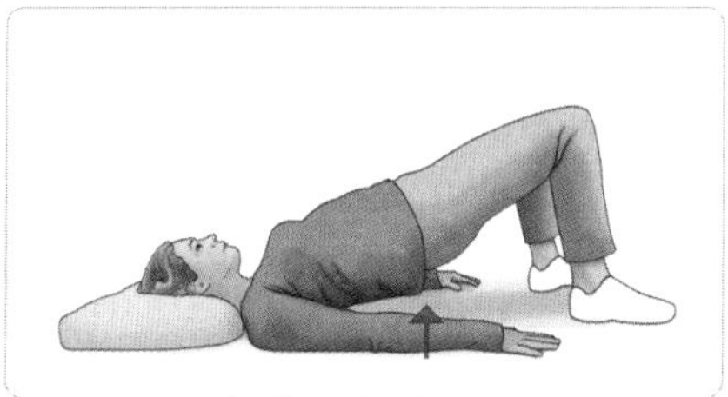

Lie on your back with both knees bent and your feet on the floor. Gently raise your buttocks off the floor 4 to 6 inches, hold for 5 seconds, and return to the starting position. Do this 5 to 10 times.

Adapted from Sports Medicine Service, Massachusetts General Hospital.

strengthen the erector spinae and abdominal muscles. None involve awkward or stressful actions that are detrimental to back muscles.

In contrast, some activities carry a relatively high risk for back injury because they involve extension, lifting, or impact. Such risky activities include football, tennis, gymnastics, wrestling, weight lifting, rowing (crew), running, aerobic dance, and ballet. Other unnatural motions that could induce pain include back arching (during gymnastics and diving), twisting (while hitting a golf ball, swinging at a baseball, or rolling a bowling ball), vertical jolting (while riding a horse), and stretching your legs strenuously (when hiking or when balancing a sailboat during a race).

If you want to continue with one of these sports following a back problem, try it—but be careful. It is helpful to work with a physical therapist to guide your return to full activity.

Complementary therapies

People with back pain often turn to complementary therapies to augment traditional medical treatments. Studies have shown that some of these therapies can help speed recovery from acute back pain, especially when combined with an exercise program. Certain therapies have also been shown to reduce painful flare-ups in people with chronic back pain. The latest treatment guidelines by the American College of Physicians (ACP) support the use of various complementary therapies for back pain, including spinal manipulation (chiropractic care), massage, acupuncture, tai chi, yoga, and meditation (see "The mind-body connection," page 31). The ACP acknowledges that the evidence for complementary therapies is generally limited, but the potential for harm is small, so there is little risk in trying them to see if you derive a benefit.

It is not entirely clear why some of these approaches help. It may be that activities such as yoga and tai chi help in multiple ways. They aid in stretching and strengthening muscles and train you to be more efficient in your motions—and thus less likely to pull your back out of whack. They also help calm and center your mind, giving you a greater sense of control over your life and over your back pain.

If you try a complementary therapy, make sure to discuss it first with the clinician treating your back condition and find a trained and experienced practitioner who is well versed in your type of back problem.

Chiropractic care

Spinal manipulation is a popular therapy for back pain. It is most often performed by chiropractors, although it may also be done by osteopaths and orthopedists. Spinal manipulation therapists apply pressure directly to one or more vertebrae using a finger or the palm of the hand. Most manipulations also involve indirect force: the practitioner carefully twists the patient's head, shoulders, and hips, temporarily displacing parts of the spine. When treating people with low back pain, chiropractors commonly also use a variety of other interventions, including massage, heat and cold therapies, and electrotherapies, as well as advice about nutrition, exercise, and other lifestyle choices.

Does chiropractic care work? Some people who use spinal manipulation therapy swear by it. They say it relieves their acute back pain and gets them on their feet faster. On the other hand, research on the effectiveness of chiropractic therapy has not always shown an advantage compared with just waiting for the problem to resolve on its own. For instance, the most recent reviews of randomized trials by the Cochrane Collaboration found that spinal manipulation for acute or chronic back pain was not clearly better than usual care (rest, pain relievers, physical therapy, etc.) in reducing pain and helping people to keep functioning.

Chiropractic manipulation carries a small degree of risk, especially for people with neck pain. Very rarely, chiropractic manipulations can worsen or even cause disc herniation and nerve-root irritation. And people with rheumatoid arthritis should avoid chiropractic care because they are more likely to experience complications. The best candidates for chiropractic manipulation are people who have no sign of nerve impairment. For them, chiropractic care tends to be satisfying and effective for acute low back pain.

If you do try spinal manipulation, always receive treatment from an experienced practitioner. And until there is more evidence, a short-term approach is best. If you don't experience considerable improvement after about six spinal manipulations, additional treatments aren't likely to be of much benefit.

Acupuncture

Acupuncture is one of the best-known and oldest alternative healing practices. It can be used to relieve or treat many types of physical pain and dysfunction. Extremely thin sterilized needles, sometimes electrified by a low-voltage power source, are inserted for brief periods at precise points along a complex network of body pathways called meridians, characterized as lines of energy that encircle the body like global lines of longitude and latitude.

Does acupuncture work? Acupuncture is subject to a strong placebo effect, whereby the expectation of benefit tends to be confirmed with self-reported pain relief. When back pain sufferers feel better, is it the acupuncture or the belief that led to the improve-

ment? That's hard to test, because sticking little needles into people is hard to fake, making it difficult to provide a placebo to test the real thing against. However, in one analysis that pooled the results of 29 past studies involving nearly 18,000 participants with back pain and other musculoskeletal problems, acupuncture relieved pain by about 50% over all. That is comparable to the relief that many people get from pain medication, suggesting that the relief provided by acupuncture may be more than just the placebo effect.

If you want to try acupuncture, be sure to choose a licensed acupuncturist. This can reduce the chance of harmful effects. The most frequently reported complication of acupuncture is infection from needles that have not been properly sterilized. Most states require a license to practice acupuncture. If you live in a state that does not require a license, choose a practitioner who is licensed in another state or is certified by the National Certification Commission for Acupuncture and Oriental Medicine (see "Resources," page 51).

Be aware, however, that acupuncture may not be reimbursed by your health plan. The typical cost of a session ranges from $65 to $125. Private insurers usually don't pay for it, nor do Medicare and Medicaid. A handful of plans may reimburse for treatment by physician-acupuncturists.

Therapeutic massage

As alternative therapies have gained popularity, many people with low back pain are turning to therapeutic massage. Massage therapists sometimes work in cooperation with orthopedic clinics or other facilities, or they may operate entirely independently.

Does therapeutic massage work? Published research provides limited guidance on how effective massage is for chronic back pain and for whom it works best. A Cochrane Collaboration review in 2015 of 25 randomized controlled studies found limited evidence for short-term relief of back pain from therapeutic massage.

The cost of a massage is covered by some health insurance plans if prescribed by a doctor. Massage therapists often have certifications to practice in their home state. (See "Resources," page 51, for information on finding a licensed massage therapist.)

Transcutaneous electrical nerve stimulation (TENS)

This therapy, which involves applying electrical stimulation to the body, is thought to provide pain relief by stimulating the release of endorphins. TENS has been around for many years, and now you can even buy your own TENS machine online.

Does TENS work? Studies on TENS as a treatment for low back pain have mostly been mixed, inconclusive, or negative. As a result, though TENS may have a pain-relieving effect for some users, guidelines from the American Academy of Neurology indicate that the technique does not help long-term back pain. The latest ACP treatment guidelines also decline to endorse TENS as a therapy for back pain.

Ultrasound therapy

Physical therapy clinics routinely offer ultrasound therapy. The therapist uses a device called a transducer to apply ultrasound energy to your sore back. Ultrasound has a warming effect on the tissues, and this could hypothetically boost blood flow in the injured area and aid recovery.

Does ultrasound therapy work? A Cochrane review pub-lished in 2014 found no convincing evidence that ultrasound is an effective treatment for reducing pain or improving general quality of life. These reviewers could find only seven randomized controlled trials of ultrasound, a limited base of evidence on which to make treatment decisions.

However, like manual massage, ultrasound appears to be harmless and some people report that it relieves discomfort. If your health plan pays for the service, there is little downside in trying it.

Complementary exercise programs

Some people with chronic back pain benefit from incorporating yoga, tai chi, or other nontraditional exercise programs into a traditional treatment regimen.

Yoga. There are many "schools" of yoga and many variations offered. What they have in common is that they involve assuming various poses (asanas), as well as practicing breathing techniques (pranayama) and achieving a meditative mental focus. The stretching and strengthening that yoga offers can help, as can the meditative mental state.

Research has found that yoga, if done with care, may offer benefits to people with chronic back problems. It reduces pain and disability, and it provides comparable relief to conventional back stretching and strengthening exercises. A 2017 review of 12 clinical trials involving a total of 1,080 people found that yoga moderately improves pain and disability over three to six months, compared with no exercise at all. However, the review concluded, it's still unclear whether yoga is better than other exercise regimens.

Safety is an issue for new practitioners of yoga and those with back pain or other musculoskeletal conditions. If you try yoga, find a teacher who has experience working with people who have back pain. In fact, some yoga classes are tailored specifically for back pain sufferers (see Figure 8, at left). Overdoing yoga can and does lead to injuries, so don't push yourself beyond your limits.

Practicing yoga for several months should show you whether

Figure 8: Adjustments to classic yoga poses

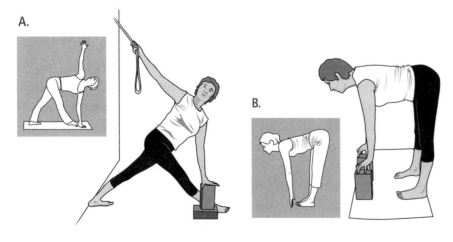

Certain types of yoga, such as Iyengar yoga, use blocks, belts, and other props to help students perform classic yoga poses such as those shown in the gray inserts above: parivrtta trikonasana, or the revolved triangle pose **(A)**, and ardha uttanasana, or the standing half forward bent pose **(B)**. Instructions are individualized, with adjustments made for age, experience, body type, physical condition, and medical problems.

it will help or not in your case. At the very least, it can be a pleasurable social activity. It may be available free or at low cost to older adults at senior centers and through adult education programs. Some for-profit yoga centers offer brief free trial classes to help you see if this activity is a good fit.

Tai chi. Tai chi is an ancient Chinese practice that incorporates slow turning movements, weight shifts, and deep breathing. It is designed to engage and benefit all parts of the body—not just the musculoskeletal system. Tai chi's benefits to overall health and well-being have been well documented in a number of populations, especially the elderly, with improvements shown in balance, muscle tone, flexibility, and bone density. A randomized controlled trial of tai chi for back pain published in 2011—the first of its kind—found that participants reported less pain and disability after 10 weeks of regular tai chi (a total of 18 40-minute sessions).

As with yoga, tai chi is low-risk and stands to help you in various ways, so there is little harm in trying it. Some community centers host "drop in" tai chi groups at public spaces and parks. Classes are also widely available. It is a relaxing and social activity, which can be a helpful mood-lifter for anyone living with chronic pain.

Alexander technique and Pilates. Other exercise programs that may help include the Alex-

The mind-body connection

The mind has a powerful influence over the body. Mind-body therapies can help some people to control pain or live with it better. The following are the more common therapies that can help when used in conjunction with other treatments.

Cognitive behavioral therapy (CBT). This form of "talk therapy" teaches people to modify how they think, feel, and behave in response to chronic pain. The goals are to lessen your perception of how bad the pain is and improve your ability to cope with it. The recommended eight to 20 treatment sessions should be done with a therapist trained in this approach. However, finding a specialist trained in CBT may be difficult in some areas. Practitioners are experimenting with telephone-based CBT using prerecorded feedback from therapists, which could make CBT available to a larger number of people.

Relaxation. Some research shows that relaxation techniques, such as progressive muscle relaxation, can lessen the subjective feeling of pain in people with chronic pain or postsurgical pain.

Deep breathing. Focusing on conscious, controlled breathing is a staple technique in relaxation. This induces what has been called a "relaxation response" that counteracts the stress response to chronic pain and may lessen its severity.

Meditation. Like focused breathing, the meditative state is a building block for many relaxation therapies. Research has shown that people who meditate regularly have a reduced subjective perception of the intensity of their pain.

Mindfulness-based stress reduction. This approach combines mindfulness meditation and yoga. A randomized controlled trial in *JAMA* in 2016 found that it was just as effective as CBT for relieving chronic low back pain.

ander technique and Pilates. Although they are not medically accredited programs, these approaches have been found in a limited number of studies to be potentially helpful for people with chronic low back pain, when conducted by a trained, experienced instructor. A Cochrane review of Pilates found moderate evidence that it reduces pain and disability, although it was unclear whether Pilates was better than other forms of exercise. As with any exercise program, improper or excessive activity can make back pain worse.

Motor control exercise. This form of therapy aims to retrain the core muscles of the lumbar spine to support the back at rest, at work, and at play. There is little evidence that it is more effective for back pain than any other type of exercise. Physical therapists provide this service.

The value of healthy living
A recurring back problem may be a message telling you to examine aspects of your lifestyle that might be contributing to the problem. Maintaining a healthy weight and

not smoking lead the list of lifestyle factors that can help your back.

Maintain a healthy weight

Although carrying too much weight is not proven to cause back pain conditions in the first place, being overweight or obese can slow your recovery from back trouble. Those extra pounds also increase the risk that back pain will return.

The heavier you are, the greater the load your spine must carry. To make matters worse, if the bulk of your weight comes in the form of abdominal fat, rather than muscle, your center of gravity can shift forward. This shift puts added pressure on your back. By maintaining a healthy weight, you can ease the burden on your spine.

To see if you are at a healthy (normal) weight, calculate your body mass index (BMI). This measure takes both your height and weight into consideration. You can find a BMI calculator online, at www.health.harvard.edu/bmi. Not only will you help your back if you maintain a normal BMI (in the range of 19 to 25), but you'll also lower your risk for many diseases, including heart attack, stroke, type 2 diabetes, and high blood pressure.

Kick the habit

You've undoubtedly heard this message before: smoking harms your health. Not only does it raise your risks for lung cancer, heart disease, hypertension, and other serious health problems, but it also jeopardizes your back.

Research shows that smokers have more frequent episodes of back pain than nonsmokers, and the more people smoke, the higher the risk of such episodes, according to one study. Nicotine is toxic to the intervertebral discs, contributing to low back pain in two ways. First, nicotine hampers the flow of blood to the vertebrae and discs. This impairs their function and may trigger a bout of back pain. Second, smokers tend to lose bone faster than nonsmokers, putting them at greater risk for osteoporosis, another common cause of back pain (see "Osteoporotic fractures," page 14).

Lighten your load

Backpacks have become ubiquitous—at school, at work, at play. But an overstuffed backpack can lead to back trouble.

Most orthopedic doctors have long recognized that backpacks increase the risk of certain types of back pain, especially in students. A survey by the American Academy of Orthopaedic Surgeons found that nearly 60% of the doctors responding had treated students complaining of back and shoulder pain caused by heavy backpacks. Hauling an overloaded backpack can also cause muscle fatigue and strain and encourage the wearer to bend forward unnaturally. Heavy messenger bags can similarly exacerbate back pain.

If you (or a child or grandchild) use a backpack, use both

Figure 9: The laws of lifting

Follow these basic steps whenever you need to lift something:

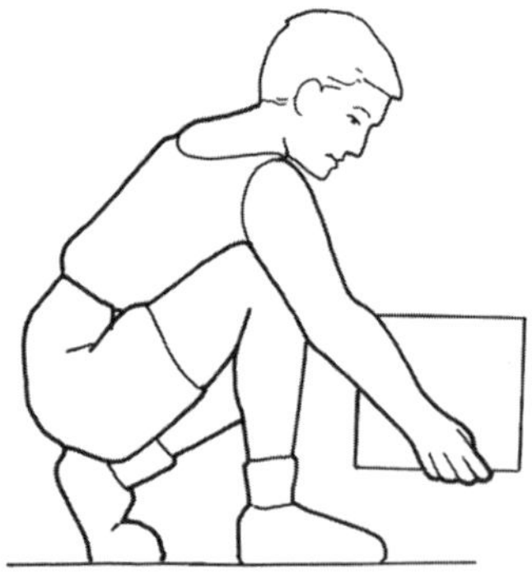

- Face the object and position yourself close to it.
- Bend at your knees, not your waist, and squat down as far as you comfortably can.
- Tighten your stomach and keep your buttocks tucked in.
- Lift with your legs, not your back muscles.
- Don't try to lift the object too high. Don't raise a heavy load any higher than your waist; keep a light load below shoulder level.
- Keep the object close to you as you lift it.
- If you need to turn to set something down, don't twist your upper body. Instead, turn your entire body, moving your shoulders, hips, and feet at the same time.
- Ask for help with lifting anything that's very heavy.

the pack's straps instead of slinging one strap over a shoulder. Try to carry only the essentials, and lighten your load whenever possible. Opt for backpacks that have different-sized compartments to help distribute weight evenly. And look for wide, padded straps and a padded back. A strap that fastens around the hips can also redistribute pressure away from the spine and place it on the hips instead.

When carrying a heavy load, put the heaviest items as close as possible to the center of the back, and use the hip strap for support. For very heavy loads, use a backpack with wheels and wheel it rather than wearing it whenever possible. Above all, remember to bend from your knees when picking up your pack (see Figure 9, page 32).

Develop back-healthy habits

Everyday activities, from vacuuming to sitting in front of a computer for hours, can take a toll on your back, particularly if you aren't schooled in proper body mechanics. You can take some of the pressure off your back by following these simple tips:

- While standing to perform ordinary tasks like chopping vegetables or folding laundry, keep one foot on a small step stool.
- When sitting, keep your knees a bit higher than your hips and bend them at a 90-degree angle. Sit with your feet comfortably on the floor. If your feet don't

Don't rely on a back belt

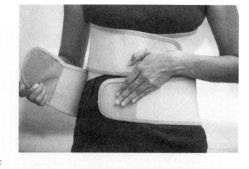

Once worn only by weight lifters, back belts have gained popularity among workers who must often lift goods—from grocery store clerks to airline baggage handlers. With back problems accounting for nearly 20% of all workplace injuries, and annual costs in the billions, it's no surprise that some companies require their workers to use these belts.

But studies have cast doubt on whether these belts help protect workers' backs or reduce sick time and workers' compensation claims. A recent randomized clinical trial found no advantage from wearing a back belt and getting training in safe lifting versus training alone or general exercise.

The National Institute of Occupational Safety and Health (NIOSH) says there is no definitive scientific evidence that back belts either prevent injuries or not. Nor is it clear whether belts decrease the force exerted on the spine, or whether they serve as a reminder to lift properly (see Figure 9, page 32). On the contrary, NIOSH has expressed concern that these belts may do harm by giving workers a false sense of security. According to NIOSH, some workers think they can lift heavier items when wearing the belts, which could lead to more—not fewer—injuries. As a result, the agency doesn't recommend employers insist that their workers use back belts to prevent back injuries.

reach the floor, put a book or a small stool under them.

- Choose an office chair that offers good back support (preferably with an adjustable backrest, lumbar support, armrests, and wheels), and set up your work space so you don't have to do a lot of twisting.
- Don't remain sitting or standing in the same position for too long. Stretch, shift your position, or take a short walk when you can.
- Because vacuuming can take a toll on your back, tackle rooms in chunks, spending no more than five to 10 minutes at a time doing this task.
- Try not to overload briefcases

or backpacks (see "Lighten your load," page 32).

- Make frequent stops when driving long distances.
- While driving, sit back in your seat, and if your seat does not provide sufficient lumbar support, place a rolled blanket or some towels behind your lower back. Try to shift your weight occasionally. If you have cruise control, use it when you can. Also consider using a foam seat cushion to absorb some of the vibration.
- Sleep on your side if you can, and bend your knees toward your chest a bit. Also, choose a pillow that keeps your head level with

Gentle exercises for neck pain

Perform these movements to the point where you feel a slight stretch but no pain. Note: While these exercises are fine for most people with neck problems, do not do them if you have a fracture or a recent, significant neck injury, or when movement exacerbates the pain. Check with your doctor if you've had a recent neck trauma or if you're not sure you should exercise your neck.

▼ Neck stretching

These stretches help relieve tight neck muscles. At the same time, they reduce compression of the vertebrae caused by such tension, and they help maintain or extend the neck's range of motion.

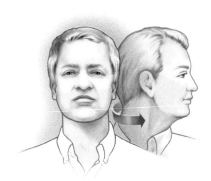

Rotation range-of-motion

Start by facing forward. Turn your head slowly to one side. Hold 3 seconds and return to the original position. Turn your head slowly to the other side. Hold 3 seconds and return to the original position. Repeat 10 times.

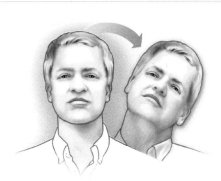

Side bending range-of-motion

Face forward and let your head bend slowly to the side. Hold 3 seconds and repeat to the other side. Repeat 10 times. Do this exercise slowly and gently. For an additional stretch, when your head is bent to the side, let it roll slowly forward about 45 degrees and hold it there for 3 seconds.

Note: Physical therapists Nancy Capparelli and Tina Nebhnani of Beth Israel Deaconess Medical Center in Boston helped design this program.

▼ Neck strengthening

Strengthening the muscles surrounding the cervical spine alleviates some of the pressure on the facet joints. It also helps maintain proper alignment of the spine, which in turn reduces muscle strain on the surrounding areas.

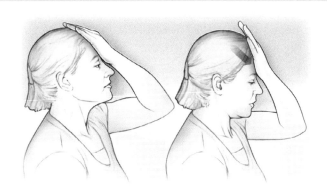

Front neck muscles:

This exercise can be done in a sitting position—at the office, for example—or lying down with your knees bent and feet flat on the floor. Place your palm on your forehead and press gently as you try to bring your chin to your chest; your neck muscles will tighten without your head moving. Hold for a count of 3 to 5 seconds. Repeat 10 times, twice daily.

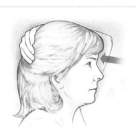

Rear neck muscles:

Place one or both hands behind your head and use them to resist as you press your head backward. Hold for a count of 3 to 5. Repeat 10 times, twice daily.

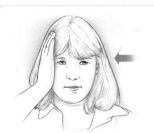

Side neck muscles:

Place your right palm on the right side of your head, using it to resist as you try to bend your right ear toward your shoulder. Hold for a count of 10. Repeat on the left.

Rotation muscles (not shown):

Place your right hand on the right side of your head. Try to rotate your head to the right, resisting with your hand. Hold for a count of 3 to 5. Repeat on the left. Repeat 10 times.

your spine; your pillow shouldn't prop your head up too high or let it droop. Choose a mattress that's firm enough to support your spine (so that it doesn't sag into the bed) and that follows your body's contours (see "Ask the doctor: What type of mattress is best for people with low back pain?" on page 25).

Safeguard your neck

Like your back, your neck is vulnerable to aches and pains. Neck pain can be brought on by a variety of triggers, including strains, sprains, muscle tension, poor posture (especially when working at a computer), sleeping on a pillow that's too high or too low, and stress. To prevent neck pain, the following tips can help.

Keep your head straight. Poor head posture can strain your neck muscles. Try to avoid having your head rest too far forward while driving or looking at a computer monitor. Move your head back so that your ear canal is aligned with the front of your shoulders. If you sleep on your side, choose a pillow that keeps your neck muscles aligned with your spine (so you could draw a straight line down the center of your head and body while resting on your side).

Get moving. Try not to sit for long periods of time. Take a break by stretching or going for a mini-walk every 20 minutes or so.

Use a headset or speaker setting. Cradling the telephone between your ear and shoulder can strain your neck. If you use the phone a lot, invest in a headset or use the speaker setting on your phone.

Keep stress in check. Managing your stress level has many health benefits, including warding off neck pain. Find a relaxation technique—such as yoga, meditation, or deep breathing—that works for you (see "The mind-body connection," page 31).

Flex your muscles. Strengthen your neck muscles by performing neck exercises every day. (For suggestions, see "Gentle exercises for neck pain," page 34.) ◢

Medications for back pain

Relieving pain is an essential part of treatment for a back condition. If you have a short-term flare-up, pain relievers can help make you more comfortable, so you can continue your work and other major activities while recovering. If you have a chronic (long-term) back condition, pain control may become a part of your daily life.

Your options for managing pain include both over-the-counter and prescription medications. Some, such as ibuprofen (Advil, Motrin) and naproxen (Aleve), are available in both forms, albeit at different doses. In general, prescription versions are stronger than over-the-counter products.

For long-term, chronic pain, you get the best results by taking the medication on a regular schedule rather than only when the pain flares up. Managing chronic pain effectively is a bit like fighting a brush fire: it's best to intervene when the problem is just smoldering. Once your symptoms ignite, it's much harder to damp them down again.

Over-the-counter pain relievers

Common over-the-counter pain relievers include acetaminophen (Tylenol) and the nonsteroidal anti-inflammatory drugs (NSAIDs) ibuprofen, naproxen, and plain old aspirin (see Table 1, below). Usually, over-the-counter options are sufficient to relieve acute (short-term) back pain. They are recommended as the first-line therapy rather than stronger drugs.

Table 1: Frequently used over-the-counter medications

GENERIC NAME (BRAND NAME)	HOW LONG DOES IT TAKE TO WORK?	HOW LONG DOES IT LAST?	MAXIMUM DAILY DOSE	COMMENTS
acetaminophen (Tylenol and others)	30 minutes	4–6 hours	3,000 mg	• Fewer gastrointestinal side effects make it useful for mild pain. • In high doses, potentially toxic to the liver and kidneys, especially in heavy drinkers. • Can be combined with opioid medications.
aspirin (Bayer, Bufferin, others)	30 minutes	4–6 hours	4,000 mg	• Inhibits blood clotting and shouldn't be used before or after surgery. Aspirin products also pose a risk of gastrointestinal discomfort and bleeding. • Drugs in the same salicylate group as aspirin—such as trisalicylate (Trilisate), diflunisal (Dolobid), and salsalate (Disalcid)—are preferred for people with stomach and bleeding problems.
ibuprofen (Advil, Motrin, others)	30 minutes	4–6 hours	2,400 mg	• Safer and better tolerated than aspirin. • Potent anti-inflammatory effect.
naproxen sodium (Aleve)	30 minutes	8–12 hours	1,100 mg	• Same pain-relieving effects as ibuprofen. • Stays in the blood longer than ibuprofen, so it needs to be taken only twice a day. • Greater risk of gastrointestinal side effects than ibuprofen.

Many people try acetaminophen because it is less likely to irritate the stomach and intestinal lining or cause gastrointestinal bleeding, as NSAIDs might. But although acetaminophen controls pain and fever, it does not reduce inflammation in strained tissues as NSAIDs do. Another problem with acetaminophen is that taking too much can damage the liver, leading to a liver transplant or death (see "Acetaminophen: Save your stomach, hurt your liver?" at right). And some studies have found that acetaminophen is not a particularly potent pain reliever for back problems.

On the other hand, acetaminophen is fairly safe when used correctly and still worth a try, since some individuals find it quite helpful. Whether you take acetaminophen or NSAIDs, don't exceed the recommended daily doses, and use the lowest dose needed to control your pain.

Prescription pain relievers

Severe back pain, such as that from a herniated disc or another nerve-compression syndrome, may require a higher level of pain relief than is possible or safe with over-the-counter medications. In such a case, your doctor can offer various prescription options, either alone or in combination, to achieve the pain control you need.

COX-2 inhibitors

A special class of NSAIDs known as COX-2 inhibitors were once promoted as "stomach-friendly" alternatives to other NSAIDs, with less risk of stomach upset or bleeding. These drugs used to include celecoxib (Celebrex), rofecoxib (Vioxx), and valdecoxib (Bextra). Both Vioxx and Bextra were subsequently withdrawn from the market after studies found that people who took COX-2 inhibitors were more likely to have heart attacks and strokes. At present, celecoxib is the only COX-2 inhibitor that is still available in the United States.

Celecoxib may be helpful to certain people with musculoskeletal pain who can't tolerate traditional NSAIDs because of gastrointestinal problems. And it may be useful for those taking anticoagulants (blood thinners), since it doesn't affect platelet function. Ask

Acetaminophen: Save your stomach, hurt your liver?

Acetaminophen (Tylenol) has been perceived as a "stomach-safe" alternative to aspirin and other non-steroidal anti-inflammatory drugs (NSAIDs). But in recent years, that perception has changed. If used improperly, acetaminophen poses serious risks to the liver even at doses once thought to be safe. According to FDA statistics, accidental and intentional acetaminophen overdoses send 56,000 people to emergency rooms every year.

To use acetaminophen safely, don't exceed the generally recommended maximum of 3,000 milligrams (mg) per day, or the amount in six "extra-strength" (500-mg) Tylenol tablets. The older standard was 4,000 mg per day, but that is no longer generally recommended for most people. Don't take more than 1,000 mg at any one time. When in doubt, ask your doctor how much acetaminophen is safe for you.

To help prevent excessive dosing, the FDA recommends that health care professionals stop prescribing or dispensing combination pain relievers that contain more than 325 milligrams (mg) of acetaminophen. Tablets containing 1,000 mg are still available over the counter but should be taken with extra caution and in consultation with your clinician.

Also, be aware that more than 600 prescription and over-the-counter products contain acetaminophen as one of their active ingredients. These medications include over-the-counter cold, flu, and sleep drugs. Read medication labels carefully, and do not exceed more than 3,000 mg per day of acetaminophen from all sources combined. If you drink alcohol on a regular basis, avoid acetaminophen altogether, since the drug is more toxic at lower doses in drinkers.

your doctor whether the heart risks are a particular concern for you.

Muscle relaxants

Muscle relaxants are sometimes prescribed to people with acute low back pain. Temporary use of muscle relaxants, taken as prescribed, can be useful for people who have severe muscle spasms following the onset of back pain. And studies show that the muscle relaxant tizanidine (Zanaflex) combined with acetaminophen or an NSAID provided more short-term pain relief than acetaminophen or an NSAID alone. The drugs can make you drowsy, though, so be careful.

Table 2: Prescription opioids for back pain

GENERIC NAME (BRAND NAME)	USUAL DOSAGE	COMMENTS
codeine (usually generic)	15–60 mg every 4 hours	• Often combined with acetaminophen. • One of the most commonly prescribed pain medications. • Has a ceiling effect: doses greater than 60 mg often have no additional painkilling benefit. • Used for mild to moderate pain resulting from a variety of causes, such as injury and surgery.
fentanyl (Duragesic patch)	Delivers tiny doses at a rate of 25–100 micrograms (mcg) per hour	• Related to meperidine (Demerol). • 75–125 times more potent than morphine for temporary pain and 30–40 times more potent for persistent pain. • Unlike morphine, does not promote histamine release, so is less likely to cause allergic reactions and other side effects. • Can be given via skin patch because it is highly fat-soluble.
hydrocodone (Lorcet, Lortab, Norco, Vicodin, Zohydro ER, others)	Variable	• Semisynthetic compound related to codeine. • Less potent painkiller compared with oxycodone. • Most formulations of hydrocodone include other painkillers, usually acetaminophen. • A newer brand, Zohydro ER (hydrocodone bitartrate), contains only hydrocodone in a time-release formulation. • Used to treat pain after injury or surgery.
hydromorphone (Dilaudid, Exalgo)	2 mg every 4–6 hours	• A derivative of morphine but about five times more potent, with a slightly shorter duration. • Oral, rectal, extended release, and injectable formulations are available.
methadone (Dolophine, Methadose)	2.5–10 mg every 3–8 hours	• Used as a maintenance drug for people addicted to opioids. Also used to treat severe pain. • Stays active in the body longer than other opioids. • Side effects, such as sedation and slowed breathing, outlast pain-relieving effects.
morphine (Kadian, Morphabond, MS Contin, Oramorph, Roxanol)	10–30 mg every 4 hours for immediate-release oral morphine, but dosages vary widely depending on route of administration; long-acting formulations last 12–24 hours	• Can be taken in many forms: by mouth, as a rectal suppository, through injection, or through catheters threaded into spaces surrounding the spinal cord. • The oral form is one-sixth to one-third as effective as other forms because the drug is metabolized in the liver. • Small amounts of morphine given through catheters in the spine can produce profound pain relief that lasts 12–24 hours. • MS Contin is a sustained-release formula created by covering morphine granules with a waxy coating. Oramorph is a liquid that can be taken by mouth. Morphabond is a new abuse-resistant formulation.
oxycodone (OxyContin, Percocet, Percodan, Roxicet, Roxicodone, Tylox, others)	Variable	• Semisynthetic compound related to codeine. • Roxicodone and OxyContin are oxycodone alone; Percodan is oxycodone combined with aspirin; Percocet, Roxicet, and Tylox are oxycodone combined with acetaminophen. • Effective when taken orally. • Used to treat pain after injury or surgery.
tramadol (ConZip, Ryzolt, Ultram)	50–100 mg every 4–6 hours; should not exceed 4,000 mg	• A semisynthetic opiate with effects and toxicities similar to other opiates. • About 15% less potent than codeine. • Usefulness as a postoperative drug still being studied.

Opioids (narcotics)

If your pain is intense and has not responded to other medications, or if you are suffering from very severe pain from a compression fracture, your doctor may give you a prescription for an opioid painkiller (also called a narcotic) for a limited period of time (see Table 2, page 38). Although narcotic pain relievers are standard tools for cancer pain and recovery from surgery, extended use to treat a chronic back problem is controversial. In the latest treatment guidelines for back pain, the American College of Physicians recommends that narcotic pain relievers should be used only when all other options are exhausted (see "Can opioid pain relievers be used safely?" on page 40).

Some doctors are reluctant to prescribe narcotic pain relievers because of concern that patients could become addicted to them. Other physicians argue that narcotics are safe in low doses and have a low risk of abuse in people with no prior history of misusing opioids—although the danger remains that people already addicted to narcotic painkillers may get hold of them and abuse them. Manufacturers have been trying to thwart abuse by developing new, tamper-resistant formulations.

Antidepressants and anticonvulsants

Back pain involves the central nervous system—which includes the brain and spinal cord—as well as the back itself. Drugs that act on the central nervous system can help people if part of their pain originates in nerves (neuropathic pain) and not just in the muscles, joints, and other musculoskeletal elements of the back.

Increasingly, certain antidepressants are prescribed for neuropathic pain. These include tricyclic antidepressants, such as amitriptyline (Elavil), doxepin (Sinequan, other brands), and nortriptyline (Aventyl, Pamelor). These drugs may interfere with pain signals on their way through the spinal cord. Other antidepressants used for chronic pain are serotonin-norepinephrine reuptake inhibitors (SNRIs), such as duloxetine (Cymbalta, other brands), milnacipran (Savella), and venlafaxine (Effexor).

Besides antidepressants, drugs called anticonvulsants also interfere with nerve pain and are being used to treat chronic back ailments. These include gabapentin (Neurontin, other brands), a drug originally developed to treat epilepsy; lamotrigine (Lamictal); carbamazepine (Carbatrol, Epitol, Tegretol); and pregabalin (Lyrica, other brands).

Figure 10: A look at two injection therapies

Epidural

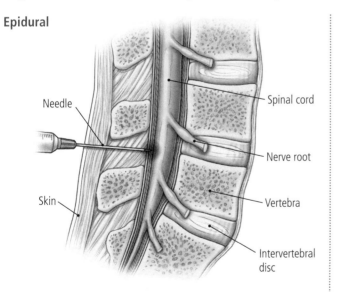

Epidural steroid injections involve the injection of steroid medications into the epidural space. This area lies outside the dura mater, a membrane that covers the spinal cord.

Facet joint

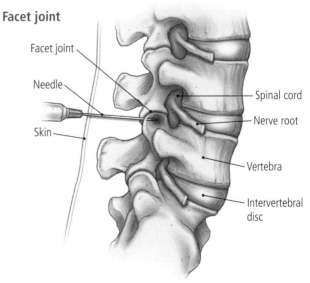

When back pain is caused by an irritated facet joint, a doctor may suggest treating the problem with an injection of a steroid combined with a local anesthetic. Known as a facet joint injection, this therapy delivers medication directly into the affected joint.

These drugs all have potential side effects—some quite serious. For example, gabapentin may be associated with an increased risk of suicide and should be used cautiously. But for people with intolerable nerve pain, drugs that act on the central nervous system can be a helpful addition to traditional painkillers.

Injection therapies

Injections of anti-inflammatory medications called corticosteroids may provide modest but temporary relief from sharp, shooting pain caused by nerve compression, such as sciatica. For people with chronic backaches, research has not shown clear benefits.

Depending on your diagnosis, injections might target the epidural space (the gap between the vertebrae and spinal cord), the lumbar discs, or the facet joints (see Figure 10, page 39). (Many women who've experienced childbirth are familiar with epidurals, in which an anesthetic is injected into the epidural space to numb pain from the waist down.) For back problems, injections are provided in an outpatient setting—for example, a doctor's office—by a specialist, such as an orthopedist, anesthesiologist, radiologist, physiatrist, or neurologist. The doctor may inject either an anesthetic, a corticosteroid, or both.

Research findings on injection therapies have been mixed. Studies show that most people with acute sciatica feel less pain and discomfort in their legs following epidural injections. However, the injections don't always relieve pain or improve a person's ability to function. Nor do they reduce the need for surgery. Thus, the epidural injection is not a cure per se, but rather a way to relieve sciatic pain while the back problem gets better on its own.

It is important to know that injection therapy involves inserting a needle into the spinal area and thus comes with risks. Serious complications are uncommon, but they include headaches caused by puncturing the sheath covering the spinal cord (the dura), infection, and bleeding. The injections themselves can be quite painful, and repeated injections of corticosteroids may raise blood sugar levels or blood pressure. These medicines are also associated with higher rates of osteoporosis.

Can opioid pain relievers be used safely?

Amid the current epidemic of opioid addiction, doctors have become more careful about prescribing opioids (narcotics) for back pain. Opioids include such drugs as hydrocodone (Vicodin), oxycodone (OxyContin), oxymorphone (Opana), methadone (Methadose), and fentanyl (Duragesic).

When taking opioids for back pain, some people may be at higher risk of addiction because of a history of substance abuse, a family history of addiction, or genetic factors. However, most people prescribed opioids for back pain for a limited time do not end up becoming addicted. Addiction involves more than just developing a physical dependence on the drug. It involves a loss of control over your daily life, despite physical, medical, and legal consequences.

Certain health care practices can help to prevent addiction. The CDC has released guidelines for doctors to help them prescribe opioids safely. These guidelines mirror other expert recommendations for treatment of chronic pain.

The "last resort" principle. First, consider nondrug therapies (such as exercise, physical therapy, and cognitive behavioral therapy) and non-opioid drugs (such as anti-inflammatories) for chronic pain.

Combine opioids with non-narcotic pain relievers to enhance pain control. These two types of drugs work differently in the body, giving the full benefits of each without a net higher risk of side effects.

Start as low as possible. When opioids are used for chronic pain, use the lowest effective dose.

Limit prescriptions. Prescribe only enough of the drug to cover the expected duration of pain.

Prescribe extended-release opioids with caution. These formulations raise the level of narcotic pain reliever in the blood gradually. But if a person doesn't get pain relief after taking one dose, he or she may be tempted to take more than directed, which is risky because the amount of narcotic in the body stays higher for a longer time. In contrast, short-acting opioids bring relief more quickly, but the effect diminishes sooner. The person may have to take pills more often, but that reduces the overall risk.

Follow up. Regularly monitor patients to make sure opioids are improving their pain and day-to-day function without causing harm. If harm outweighs benefits, step up other therapies and work with patients to taper them off opioids.

In 2012, contaminated epidural injections from one pharmacy infected hundreds of people with fungal meningitis. Such events are rare, but they remind us that no procedure comes with a safety guarantee.

Prolotherapy injections

Prolotherapy, also known as sclerotherapy, involves injecting ligaments in the spinal column with dextrose (sugar) and lidocaine (an anesthetic). This treatment remains unproven and controversial. The premise is that causing acute inflammation at the injection sites will kick-start the natural healing process and strengthen the supportive back ligaments. Prolotherapy injections are sometimes combined with other therapies, such as steroid injections, exercise, and spinal manipulation.

Studies to date on prolotherapy have found limited and short-term benefit. A review of research by the Cochrane Collaboration found no strong evidence that prolotherapy helps people with chronic back pain, and the American Pain Society recommends against it. When considering an injection therapy with weak or uncertain research backing, it pays to ask your doctor to give reasons for recommending it, given the potential dangers of injections in the spinal column. ◗

▶ Learning to live with chronic back pain

For an unfortunate few, back pain never completely disappears, despite medication and other therapies. In such cases, the goal of treatment becomes "functional restoration." This means a highly qualified team of professionals from a number of medical specialties help you learn how to continue doing the things that really matter to you.

You can get this kind of help through a back rehabilitation program, which you can typically find at specialized clinics called spine centers. Back rehab teams generally consist of a pain management physician, nurses, physical and occupational therapists, and a psychologist. As you become more physically conditioned, you may become able to do things you thought you'd never be able to do again. The focus switches from feeling hopeless to feeling hopeful.

When is surgery an option?

Surgery is helpful only under certain conditions. Your doctor will recommend immediate surgery if you have cauda equina syndrome or another "red flag" condition, such as a tumor or traumatic injury.

In the case of other conditions—such as a herniated disc, spinal stenosis, a compression fracture, or spondylolisthesis—your doctor may recommend surgery if conservative measures don't provide adequate relief after a sufficient period, usually a minimum of six weeks. To rule in favor of surgery for nerve-compression problems, such as a herniated disc, you will need to have clear evidence that the disc is compressing a nerve root. An imaging procedure, such as a CT or MRI scan, may provide that evidence. If diagnostic tests do not reveal clear signs of pressure on a particular nerve, the cause of the back pain may lie elsewhere, and surgery would therefore not be helpful.

However, outside of emergency situations, the decision to have back surgery is yours to make in conjunction with your doctor. This means that you will need to carefully consider all the risks and benefits involved. The more you know, the better, because surgery comes with substantial risks.

Weighing the risks and benefits of surgery

As with any surgery, you run the risk of infection at the site of the incision. General anesthesia carries some risks, too, but it is much safer today than in the past.

In addition, back surgery poses a small risk of serious complications. It is possible to end up with a nerve injury and experience weakness, numbness, or tingling in one or both legs. And there is the chance of bleeding from the large vessels that lie in front of the spinal discs, which can be damaged during the procedure. You can also suffer an infection of a disc or adjacent tissues, requiring prolonged antibiotics and sometimes a second operation. These serious prob-

▶ Choosing a surgeon

Choose your surgeon carefully. A good place to start is with a referral from your primary care doctor. You might also seek recommendations from people who've recently undergone successful back surgery.

Training and experience in back surgery are essential. Look for a surgeon with board certification in orthopedic surgery or neurosurgery and special training in spine surgery. (Board certification requires passing special tests to demonstrate mastery in a particular medical specialty.)

In addition, look for a surgeon who is attentive and concerned about you and takes the time to answer questions in appropriate detail. It's important to ask a surgeon about his or her experience and comfort with a specific operation, and to get a direct, candid response.

lems are rare when an experienced orthopedist or neurosurgeon performs the operation (see "Choosing a surgeon," above).

Assuming you have a non-emergency condition that is treatable with surgery, the decision whether or not to have the operation is a big one. How do you make it? One way is to answer the questions below. There are no "right" answers—only your answers.

- Do you fully understand your back problem, including the various treatment options, the evidence supporting them, and the likely outcomes of these treatments?
- Do you know the likely future course of your back condition if untreated, so you can choose between a wait-and-watch approach and surgery?
- Has the doctor explained the risks and benefits of surgery for your back problem in a way that you understand?
- Do you understand how likely the surgery is to relieve pain and reduce disability, and for how long? How likely will it be that you might need additional surgeries?
- How do you feel about taking risks of any sort?

Consider your personality, lifestyle, age, and other medical conditions.

- How do you feel about the risks associated with both the surgical and the nonsurgical treatment options for your back problem?
- How much do you value functioning at a high level, and how much risk are you willing to take to get to a higher level of function? For example, a professional athlete would most likely want more functionality and be prepared to take more risk. For other people, the stakes may not be so high.

Discuss these questions with your doctor. This will help you reach an informed decision.

Surgery for disc disease

More than 90% of people with herniated discs will recover within several months without surgery, simply by using conservative measures. But if you are among the other 10%—or if you simply don't want to wait and see what happens—surgery is an option.

Several types of procedures exist for disc surgery, which is sometimes referred to as lumbar decompression surgery because the operation relieves the pressure on the spinal nerve roots. Your surgeon can help you determine which procedure is best for you. One alternative is implantation of an artificial disc (see "What about artificial discs?" at right).

But the most common approach is discectomy, the removal of a portion of a damaged disc pressing on nerves. Results from the Spine Patient Outcomes Research Trial (SPORT) suggest that discectomies provide better pain relief over a four-year period than nonsurgical treatments. However, it's not clear whether surgery offers a greater advantage after 10 years.

Standard discectomy

A standard discectomy involves making an opening in the spinal canal between adjacent laminae (the bony plates of each vertebra that join in the midline), then removing material protruding from the abnormal disc (see Figure 11, page 44). Since the problem area is directly exposed and visible to the surgeon during the procedure, the risk of inadvertent damage to neighboring bone, ligaments, and nerve roots is minimized.

The surgeon will clear out any detached disc material (known as free fragments). If the disc has not fragmented but a significant portion protrudes into the spinal canal, the surgeon will trim the bulging portion. Some portion of the soft part of the disc between the vertebrae can also be removed.

Several different procedures may be part of the operation, including the following:

- **Laminotomy or laminectomy.** With a laminotomy, the surgeon removes a small part of the bone of the lamina. In a laminectomy, the surgeon removes the entire lamina. Removing the lamina enlarges the size of the spinal canal, thus relieving pressure on the nerves within.
- **Foraminotomy or foraminectomy.** These procedures expand the openings through which the nerve roots exit the spinal canal. A foraminectomy removes more bone and tissue than in a foraminotomy.

Standard discectomy has traditionally involved

What about artificial discs?

Damaged or diseased knee and hip joints are routinely replaced with artificial joints, so why not damaged discs, too? An artificial disc is designed to mimic a natural disc, providing normal movement between the vertebrae and maintaining the distance between them.

Spinal disc replacement has become common in some European countries, but to date, this high-tech solution for chronic pain and disability from damaged discs has not proven itself clearly superior to either spinal fusion or conventional rehabilitation. Results to date have been mixed. Although a recent review of six clinical trials found results with artificial discs as good as or better than those for lumbar fusion, an earlier review by the Cochrane Collaboration of seven randomized trials found no meaningful difference in pain relief or daily function between people who had fusion and those who got a new disc.

As with any spinal surgery, disc replacement comes with risks, too. Rare but catastrophic adverse effects of artificial disc implants include paralysis, major bleeding, and growth of new bone in the space around the artificial disc.

Keeping in mind all these caveats, artificial discs nonetheless work extremely well in some individuals. Unfortunately, at present it's hard to reliably predict who will enjoy long-lasting benefits from a spinal disc replacement.

a hospital stay of a couple of days, typically followed by physical therapy at home. But increasingly, discectomy is done on an outpatient basis in healthy people, who then can go home the same day.

Recovery is gradual. For the first six weeks or so following surgery, try not to sit for longer than 15 to 20 minutes at a time. When you do sit, recline the back of your chair about 30 degrees from vertical. Avoid bending, lifting, and twisting, but start walking as soon as you can tolerate it.

Two weeks after the operation, you can begin stationary bicycling and swimming. If you develop back or leg pain, ease off and talk with your doctor.

You can usually resume normal, nonvigorous activities six weeks after surgery, although you and your surgeon can adjust the schedule according to your individual progress. Results from the SPORT study show that people who had discectomy surgery improved somewhat more quickly than those who received usual care, and these improvements continued for at least four years.

Microdiscectomy

Microdiscectomy is a type of discectomy that involves a smaller incision than the conventional procedure. Its benefits include a shorter hospital stay and less risk of complications, such as postoperative blood clots, that can come with a longer hospitalization. However, microdiscectomy is a more technically challenging procedure and requires the use of a magnifying instrument to view the disc and nerves. Like all spinal surgery, the procedure poses some risk, such as nerve damage and infection, but these are very rare. The success rate of microdiscectomy is similar to that of standard discectomy.

Percutaneous discectomy

This minimally invasive procedure involves the removal of a portion of a damaged disc through an instrument inserted in the back. "Percutaneous" means through the skin, so the technique is, by definition, a less invasive technique than standard discectomy.

In percutaneous discectomy, the surgeon makes a tiny incision and inserts a hollow probe, about 2 millimeters (1/16 inch) in diameter. While watching on an x-ray device called a fluoroscope, the surgeon guides the probe precisely to the affected disc. The surgeon then moves the probe into the center of the disc and uses an automated cutting-irrigating-suctioning tool,

Figure 11: Standard discectomy: Surgery for a herniated disc

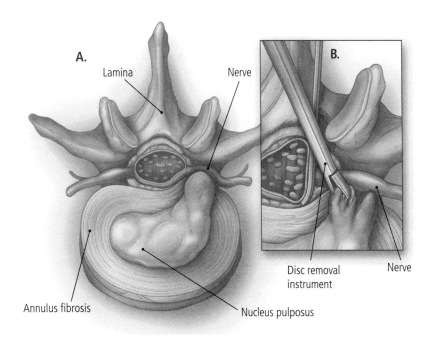

A. When a disc is herniated, the material within the disc (nucleus pulposus) bulges into the opening between vertebrae through which nerves leave the spine and extend to other parts of the body. This presses on the nerve root, causing pain.

B. During a standard discectomy, a portion of the bony arch of the vertebra (lamina) is removed. This allows the surgeon to reach and remove the disc material causing the nerve-root compression.

which is inserted through the probe, to remove some of the interior contents (nucleus) and outer shell (annulus) from the herniated disc.

This delicate operation can reduce both the pressure and volume of the material inside the disc, thus relieving pressure on the nerve root. Because the procedure involves a small incision and local anesthesia only, you can usually return home on the same day or the next. For the following few weeks, you'll need to avoid sitting for longer than 15 to 20 minutes at a time, as well as bending, twisting, and lifting.

But this procedure also has substantial disadvantages compared with standard discectomy or microdiscectomy. Since the compressed nerve root remains hidden from direct observation during the operation, the surgeon often cannot be sure that the pressure on it has been reduced or eliminated. Should a bit of the soft center of the disc slip out through the outer shell, the surgeon has no way of finding and removing it. Such a free-floating piece of disc can cause pain. In addition, there is a small risk of infection and of damage to nerves, organs, and blood vessels in the area.

As well as describing a surgical approach, percutaneous discectomy is an umbrella term for a number of other percutaneous techniques, as follows.

Laser discectomy. Instead of removing some of the disc material with a cutting-irrigating-suctioning tool, the surgeon uses a medical laser to vaporize part of the nucleus. The benefits, risks, and success rates associated with laser discectomy are equivalent to those for percutaneous discectomy.

Nucleoplasty. In this technique, the surgeon inserts a small instrument into the disc nucleus and destroys a small amount of the nucleus tissue, reducing pressure inside the disc. Nucleoplasty is a minimally invasive technique that can be done on an outpatient basis, but it isn't appropriate for people with severe disc deterioration.

Chemonucleolysis. This procedure, which is more popular in Europe than in the United States, involves injecting an enzyme (chymopapain) that dissolves a portion of the herniated disc. The treatment may trigger an allergic reaction to the enzyme used in the procedure. Reactions can range from a simple rash, itching, and localized swelling to anaphylac-

tic shock, a life-threatening condition characterized by an extremely rapid, sharp drop in blood pressure. The risk of an allergic reaction can be significantly reduced, although not eliminated, by having an allergen skin test before surgery.

Intradiscal electrothermal annuloplasty (IDET). For this technique, a surgeon inserts a hollow needle into the affected disc, threads a thin catheter through the needle, and positions the catheter along the inner wall of the disc. Heating the catheter to a high temperature cauterizes the nerve fibers in the disc, making them less sensitive. The idea is to reduce the disc-related pain a person feels. Although generally considered safe, IDET is not particularly effective, with 50% of patients unhappy with the outcome of their therapy because they continue to have pain.

Spinal fusion for disc disease

Spinal fusion is a more controversial and risky option for relieving the symptoms of damaged or diseased discs. The surgeon uses bone grafts or hardware (such as plates, screws, and wire cages) to fuse two or more vertebrae together and remove the degenerated disc that is presumably responsible for the pain (see Figure 12, page 47, and "Spinal fusion for spondylolisthesis," page 46, for more detail on the procedure). The fused vertebrae essentially become a single vertebra.

Although spinal fusion for disc-related back pain is becoming more common, doctors lack strong proof from clinical trials enabling them to predict who can really benefit from this surgery (see "Is spinal fusion overused?" on page 48). At the same time, complications from failed spinal fusions can be severe. Discuss the pros and cons with your surgeon before opting for spinal fusion. It may be wise to make sure you exhaust all other options, including intensive back rehabilitation, before undergoing this surgery.

Surgery for spinal stenosis and spondylolisthesis

Spinal stenosis—narrowing of the spinal canal—is less likely than a herniated disc to clear up without treatment. People with spinal stenosis tend to be older and often have other conditions that can make their back problems worse. This may help explain why only about 20% of people with spinal stenosis improve substantially over time without treatment. Many people eventually look to surgery in hopes of relieving their symptoms. One caveat: research suggests that about 10% to 25% of people who have surgery for their spinal stenosis have a repeat surgery within seven to 10 years.

Laminectomy for spinal stenosis

The purpose of spinal stenosis surgery is to remove structures that are pressing on the nerves and contributing to symptoms. To do this, a surgeon will perform a laminectomy (see page 43) and may also remove parts of the facet joints, along with any bony overgrowths (osteophytes, commonly known as bone spurs) and herniations. Between 65% and 75% of people treated in this way eventually obtain good to excellent results. In practical terms, that means that if their pain persists at all, it can be controlled by non-narcotic or over-the-counter medications. They can also engage in physical activity with few or no restrictions.

Spinal fusion for spondylolisthesis

Spinal stenosis usually results from degeneration of discs, ligaments, or facet joints. A series of degenerative changes, including spinal stenosis, can lead to a condition called spondylolisthesis, in which one vertebra shifts forward or backward with respect to its neighbor.

When spondylolisthesis is present, a surgeon may recommend a spinal fusion (see Figure 12, page 47) to fix the position of the vertebrae permanently and prevent future displacement. In this procedure, a surgeon fuses adjacent misaligned vertebrae. The success rate for such operations varies according to the underlying problem.

Surgeons can use any of several different methods of fusion to join two or more adjacent vertebrae. The space between the vertebrae can be bridged with a graft of bone from elsewhere in the body or from a bone bank. The graft also stimulates bone growth in the area of the fusion. In addition, metal implants—typically, pedicle screws and plates—may be secured to the vertebrae, where they serve as splints to hold the vertebrae until new bone has consolidated the grafts into a strong bony strut.

Finally, small cylindrical metal cages may be inserted into the vertebrae to work as internal splints that hold the vertebrae together while the fusion takes place. These are typically made of titanium and are about an inch long.

Following spinal fusion surgery, you might wear a brace, a cast, or neither—depending on the specifics of your operation and the surgeon's advice. It usually takes about six months for the treated bones to fuse.

Successful surgery results in a stable union of the fused vertebrae. Within four to nine months, your body replaces most of the grafted bone at the surgical site with new bone. By reducing motion in the affected area of the spine, a bone fusion relieves the pain caused by abnormal movement. After fusion, the range of spinal motion will be approximately 20% to 30% less than it was originally. However, compared with your condition before surgery, when pain most likely limited your motion, you are likely to have a greater effective range of movement, as well as freedom from chronic pain. The fusion at one level of the spine translates more force to adjacent spinal levels, putting the facet joints and discs at these adjacent levels at risk of degenerative change over time.

Surgery for compression fractures

Vertebral compression fractures due to osteoporosis mainly affect postmenopausal women. About one in four postmenopausal women has had such a fracture. The standard treatment was—and still is—to wait it out while the fractured bone heals. This process can take six weeks on average and is very painful; often, narcotic painkillers are necessary to provide relief.

Two procedures for treating vertebral fractures have emerged: vertebroplasty and kyphoplasty. Both are types of vertebral augmentation. Doctors typically perform them when a person has a fracture that causes intolerable pain but can't be treated successfully with medication.

Vertebroplasty

This technique, which was developed in France and first introduced in the United States in 1993, is done on an outpatient basis and takes less than an hour. After you receive mild sedation, the physician inserts a needle into the compressed vertebra, using an x-ray for guidance. The surgeon then injects bone cement, called methylmethacrylate, into the vertebra, filling the holes and crevices. The cement hardens in about 20 minutes, stabilizing the vertebra, creating a support that helps prevent any further collapse, and alleviating pain.

Does it work? As is often the case, the research findings are mixed. Two clinical trials comparing vertebroplasty to a sham intervention (in which sur-geons simulated the procedure but did not inject any cement) offered no clear proof that the procedure improved pain and other problems associated with spinal fractures. However, a review of several studies found that vertebroplasty reduced pain and improved daily functioning and quality of life.

Kyphoplasty

This procedure is a refinement of vertebroplasty. Like vertebroplasty, kyphoplasty aims to stabilize compressed vertebrae and relieve pain. It also offers several advantages over the original procedure: it restores the

---

Figure 12: Spinal fusion surgery for spinal stenosis

Spinal stenosis with spondylolisthesis of the lumbar spine

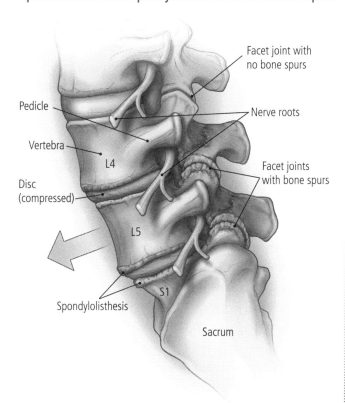

Spinal fusion surgery for stenosis

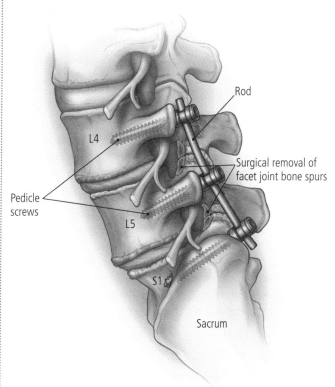

Spinal stenosis, a narrowing of the spinal canal, usually results from degeneration of the discs, the ligaments, or the facet joints on the rear part of the spine. Age-related changes can cause the discs to shrink, which reduces the space between the vertebrae and the facet joints. Stress on these joints can lead to arthritic changes, which can cause one vertebra to slip forward, a condition called spondylolisthesis. In this example, the fifth lumbar vertebra (L5) has slipped forward a few millimeters with respect to the first sacral vertebra (S1).

Surgery for spinal stenosis aims to relieve pressure on the spinal cord and nerve roots. A surgeon typically performs a laminectomy and may also remove parts of the facet joints and any bone spurs or disc herniation. To stabilize a spondylolisthesis, the surgeon inserts pedicle screws to join the vertebrae, which fixes them in place permanently. The surgeon typically also adds bone graft material to further stabilize the fusion. (The bone graft is not shown in the figure to permit a clearer view of the hardware.)

Is spinal fusion overused?

People with a variety of back conditions, not just spondylolisthesis, may be offered spinal fusion surgery. The other conditions include scoliosis, degenerative disc disease, vertebral fractures, and tumors. The number of procedures being performed, particularly for disc-related problems, has grown dramatically. Based on the most recent information, 465,000 Americans undergo fusions annually. This has left health quality experts wondering if spinal fusion procedures are being overused.

A great deal of research has focused on measuring the benefits of spinal fusion, and the results vary from study to study; they also differ for the various back conditions that are being treated. Unfortunately, there are few large clinical trials that compare spinal fusion head-to-head with more conservative treatments. Two exceptions in 2016 were a pair of studies that compared spinal fusion with simple laminectomy in people with stenosis as well as spondylolisthesis. Neither study found a benefit for fusion over laminectomy.

Large reviews of the research, pooling results from many individual studies, often find the evidence insufficient to determine whether spinal fusion surgery works better than other common options. This is typical of medical science, which is a process of continually testing options but not necessarily declaring clear winners. Often, the results of surgery in a particular study depend strongly on the severity of the back condition among the people who were recruited into the trial. What works for those people might not work for you—or it may work better.

This leaves doctors and their patients without clear-cut guidance on fusion surgery. In the end, your best move is to press your doctor for information, based on his or her experience. Ask how well it could turn out in the best-case scenario. Or, perhaps more important, ask how poorly it could turn out in the worst case. As with most medical procedures, the decision requires individual choice.

height of previously compressed vertebrae, reduces spinal deformity, and minimizes the risk of cement leakage.

Kyphoplasty takes less than an hour, although you may need to remain in the hospital overnight. After you receive mild sedation, the physician inserts a small tube-like instrument into the affected vertebra, using a special viewing instrument called a fluoroscope as a guide. Once the instrument is correctly placed, a balloon is inserted and inflated, creating a cavity in the

bone. The balloon is then deflated, and the physician injects surgical cement into the cavity. Creating such a cavity reduces the risk that the cement will leak and also pushes the vertebral endplates apart, thus restoring some height.

The research on kyphoplasty, as for vertebroplasty, is mixed. One review of past studies found no evidence of benefit from either vertebroplasty or kyphoplasty.

Know the risks

As with all invasive procedures, repairing cracked vertebrae with these techniques is not risk-free. Complications are uncommon but could include bleeding, infection, and nerve damage. If bone cement leaks from the treated area into the bloodstream or spinal canal, serious problems can occur. Also, physically shoring up one collapsed disc could increase the risk that adjacent ones will give way. The FDA has received reports of serious adverse events associated with these procedures, such as soft tissue damage, nerve-root pain and compression, pulmonary embolism, and lung or heart failure.

Surgeries for other back problems

Other back problems that may benefit from prompt surgery include infections, tumors, and certain kinds of fractures. In these situations, timely surgery is essential. In other situations—notably when surgery is recommended to cut or destroy nerves to control pain—it's best to be skeptical, since the benefits may not materialize.

Infections

If an infection is causing your back pain and antibiotics haven't been completely effective, surgery may be necessary. In an operation usually called a debridement, the surgeon removes pus and the infected and dead parts of the bone. The surgeon then washes out the affected area with a sterile solution containing antibiotics to kill the bacteria or fungi that are causing the infection. A bone fusion is also recommended when large portions of one or more vertebrae must be taken out to control the infection. Antibiotics are needed for several weeks after surgery.

Tumors

For a bone tumor originating in the spine, surgery may or may not be useful, depending on various factors. For example:

- Is the growth malignant?
- Can it be treated by radiation or chemotherapy?
- Is it making the spine unstable and vulnerable to fracture?
- Is it compressing the spinal canal or nerve roots?
- Is it located in a part of the spine where surgical removal is possible?

If the goal of an operation is to cure a cancer, the entire tumor must be removed, along with a portion of healthy bone. When the spine is weakened from the surgical removal of bone or the destruction of bone by the tumor, the weakened area must be stabilized. This is usually done with metal implants, sometimes supplemented by bone cement or bone grafts.

For cancerous tumors that have spread to the spine from another site—such as the breast—radiation, surgery, chemotherapy, or some combination of these treatment options is used, as appropriate.

Some tumors, including lipomas, teratomas, ependymomas, and neurofibromas, arise directly from the spinal cord or the nerve roots. Although rare, such growths are often painful. Whether a surgical approach is possible depends on the type of tumor, as well as its size and location.

Dislocations and vertebral fractures

Slightly displaced spinal fractures or dislocations usually heal without causing severe pain or spinal instability. Surgery is generally reserved for serious ligament and bone damage. Your doctor will determine the extent of the damage through a physical examination and analysis of imaging studies, such as MRI scans.

During an operation, the surgeon can, if necessary, remove bone fragments from the spinal canal and can implant metal plates or rods—either temporarily or permanently—to stabilize the spine and maintain its alignment during healing. Spinal fusion is usually needed to reconstruct or substitute for damaged vertebrae or ligaments, or both. ▼

Recovering from back pain

After an episode of back pain, whatever the treatment, it's essential to properly time your return to normal activities. Too rapid a return is likely to precipitate a relapse, but too timid a return can delay—or even prevent—recovery. If you are recovering from back pain, seek detailed information from your doctors about what you can do and when. Ask whether physical therapy might be helpful.

The guidelines for recuperation after surgery depend on the operation you have undergone. Your surgeon will help you work out a program for recovery, which typically includes physical therapy. Pain medications are usually very helpful in the first few days. It's vital to be out of bed, sitting up, and walking as soon as possible, although you should resume exercise and increase activities gradually. Talk to your doctor about the specific timetable that is right for you.

▶ Sex and your aching back

It's not uncommon for backaches to interfere with an individual's lovemaking. Often, people are reluctant to talk with their doctor about how their back pain affects their sexual activity. But if you find that backaches—or fears of reinjuring your back—put a damper on your sex life, ask your doctor for advice.

Here are a few suggestions that might also be helpful:

- Talk openly with your partner about your concerns.
- Avoid positions that hurt.
- Try positions that are easier on your back, such as lying on your side with your hips and your knees slightly bent.
- Be judicious and gentle. If your back is bothering you, don't aim for long, vigorous, gymnastic lovemaking.
- Try making love in the water. This can take some of the stress off your back, because water is buoyant and offers support.
- Be patient. Don't try to resume sex too soon after having a backache. If you find that your back hurts when you resume sexual activity, wait a few days before trying again.

Five rules for a safe comeback

The following are a few general principles for safe and effective recovery.

1. Let symptoms be your guide. As a general rule, avoid doing anything that hurts. If there is pain, stop the activity.

2. Increase activities gradually, according to tolerance. For example, you might start by doing four or five repetitions of an abdominal exercise, three times a day. If this doesn't cause your pain to worsen, you can increase the number of repetitions every few days—and add new exercises—as tolerated. If the exercises increase your discomfort, they can be cut back for a while, then resumed and again gradually increased. You can usually resume sexual activity once you're up and walking with minimal discomfort (see "Sex and your aching back," below left).

3. Avoid twisting your trunk or making sudden off-balance movements. Try to rid your house of clutter that can trip you up. Slippery surfaces and throw rugs are notorious for causing falls. Activities such as diving and swimming in surf can cause problems, as can lifting objects while your body is in an awkward position.

4. Exercise regularly. Appropriate exercise—such as swimming, walking, or bicycle riding (either stationary or regular)—should become an established part of your regular exercise routine.

5. Keep up good habits even after your discomfort is gone. During an episode of low back pain, a person typically moves cautiously, bending the knees when picking something up, carrying objects close to the body to minimize leverage on the back, and sitting down and getting up with care. To some extent, such back-saving maneuvers—as well as any back exercise program started in time of need—should become lifelong habits, whether or not you're concerned about impending pain. Practices such as these can help minimize the frequency of back woes. ♥

Resources

Organizations

American Academy of Orthopaedic Surgeons
9400 W. Higgins Road
Rosemont, IL 60018
847-823-7186
www.aaos.org

This nonprofit organization informs the public about orthopedics, including information on the causes, treatment, and prevention of back pain. Free fact sheets and brochures are available online. The website includes a surgeon locator.

American Academy of Physical Medicine and Rehabilitation
9700 W. Bryn Mawr Ave., Suite 200
Rosemont, IL 60018
847-737-6000
www.aapmr.org

This professional organization for physiatrists (doctors who specialize in physical medicine and rehabilitation) provides information on a variety of conditions such as low back and neck pain, spinal cord and brain injuries, osteoporosis, and arthritis. The website includes a physician locator.

American Massage Therapy Association
500 Davis St., Suite 900
Evanston, IL 60201
877-905-0577 (toll-free)
www.amtamassage.org

This organization promotes the art, science, and practice of massage therapy and provides a free locator for licensed massage therapists at www.findamassagetherapist.org or 888-THE-AMTA (888-843-2682; toll-free).

American Physical Therapy Association
1111 N. Fairfax St.
Alexandria, VA 22314
800-999-2782 (toll-free)
www.apta.org

This national professional organization for physical therapists provides links to related sites. The website includes a physical therapist locator.

National Center for Complementary and Integrative Health
National Institutes of Health
9000 Rockville Pike
Bethesda, MD 20892
888-644-6226 (toll-free)
www.nccih.nih.gov

This government agency provides science-based information on the safety and efficacy of complementary and alternative therapies. NCCIH does not provide medical advice for individuals.

National Certification Commission for Acupuncture and Oriental Medicine
76 S. Laura St., Suite 1290
Jacksonville, FL 32202
904-598-1005
www.nccaom.org

This nonprofit organization, accredited by the National Commission for Certifying Agencies, seeks to promote nationally recognized standards of competency and safety in acupuncture, Chinese herbology, and Oriental bodywork therapy.

Spine-health
790 Estate Drive, Suite 250
Deerfield, IL 60015
847-607-8577
www.spine-health.com

This commercial website provides in-depth information on back pain, including common causes, diagnostic measures, treatments, and surgery. The site also features information on recent advances. Medical professionals review all content.

Books

Heal Your Aching Back
Jeffrey N. Katz, M.D., and Gloria Parkinson
(McGraw-Hill, 2007)

This comprehensive guide to back pain, co-authored by the medical editor of this Special Health Report, covers such topics as diagnosing your problem, controlling your pain, traditional and complementary treatments, and ways to maintain a healthy back after an episode of back pain.

Yoga for Back Pain
Loren Fishman, M.D., and Carol Ardman
(W. W. Norton & Company, 2012)

Dr. Loren Fishman, a rehabilitation specialist at Columbia University's College of Physicians and Surgeons (and a practicing yogi), describes yoga poses that can help prevent back pain, relieve the pain caused by various back conditions, and promote calm to help endure any remaining pain.

Harvard Special Health Reports

The following Special Health Reports from Harvard Medical School can be ordered by calling 877-649-9457 (toll-free) or online at www.health.harvard.edu.

An Introduction to Tai Chi
Peter M. Wayne, Ph.D., Medical Editor
(Harvard Medical School, 2017)

This report provides basic tai chi moves that have been tested in studies and shown to help improve various measures of health.

An Introduction to Yoga
Sat Bir Singh Khalsa, Ph.D., and Lauren E. Elson, M.D., Medical Editors
(Harvard Medical School, 2016)

This report presents a basic yoga program that can help improve your strength, balance, and flexibility, while also promoting mindfulness and greater well-being.

Neck Pain
Robert H. Shmerling, M.D., Medical Editor
(Harvard Medical School, 2016)

This report details types of neck pain and the steps you can take to help resolve your pain. A special section focuses on preventing further pain with ergonomics, tips for safe exercise, and more.

Glossary

ankylosing spondylitis: An inflammatory disease of the spine that often leads to pain and stiffness of the back.

annulus fibrosus: The multilayered, fibrous outer portion of an intervertebral disc.

articular processes: The two upper and two lower bony projections on the back part of each vertebra that form the facet joints.

bone scan: A diagnostic procedure in which radioactive material is injected into the patient's bloodstream to produce images of the skeleton. Used to locate areas of rapid bone formation that might signal, for example, a tumor or an infection.

cauda equina: The bundle of nerve fibers that starts at the top of the small of the back and continues to the bottom of the spinal canal. The name comes from the Latin term for a horse's tail.

computed tomography (CT): A diagnostic technique in which x-rays are taken from many different directions. A computer synthesizes the x-rays to generate cross-sectional and other images of the body.

discectomy: The surgical removal of all or part of an intervertebral disc.

discitis: Inflammation or infection of an intervertebral disc.

electromyography: A series of diagnostic procedures that involve measuring electrical activity in muscles to help diagnose neuromuscular disorders.

facet joint: Any of the joints between the interlocking vertebrae that form the spine.

herniated disc: Displacement of some portion of the disc out of its normal location.

iliopsoas muscles: The two muscles that are attached to each side of the lumbar vertebrae, the inside of the pelvis, and the thighbone.

intervertebral foramina: The two narrow spaces between adjacent vertebrae (one on each side), through which nerve roots pass (singular: foramen).

kyphoplasty: A minimally invasive procedure to alleviate pain from spinal compression fractures. A balloon-like structure is placed in the affected vertebra and is inflated; the resulting cavity is filled with bone cement to stabilize the vertebral fracture.

lamina: One of the two thin, plate-like parts of each vertebra that join in the midline and form the base of the spinous process of that vertebra.

laminectomy: An operation to remove all or a portion of one or both laminae, to provide access to the spinal canal or to decompress the spinal cord and nerve roots.

lumbar spine: The five lowermost vertebrae of the spine.

magnetic resonance imaging (MRI): A diagnostic technique in which radio waves generated in a strong magnetic field are used to provide information about the tissues within the body; a computer uses this information to produce images of the tissues in many different planes.

myelography: A diagnostic technique in which x-rays are taken of the spine after a contrast medium has been injected into the space within the sheath that surrounds the spinal cord and the cauda equina.

nucleus pulposus: The gel-like central portion of an intervertebral disc.

osteophyte: A bony outgrowth, or spur, on the margin of a joint or intervertebral disc.

percutaneous discectomy: The removal of part of an intervertebral disc by means of a narrow probe inserted through the skin and muscle of the back.

processes: The seven bony projections from each vertebra, some of which mesh with similar structures on the vertebrae immediately above and below.

sciatica: Pain along the course of the sciatic nerve (from the buttock, down the back and side of the leg, and into the foot and toes), often because of a herniated disc.

spinal fusion: A procedure to join two or more vertebrae with a bone graft, and often with screws and plates, in order to eliminate motion and relieve pain.

spinal stenosis: A narrowing of the spinal canal, which can result in compression of nerve roots.

spinous process: The lever-like backward projection from each vertebra, to which muscles and ligaments are attached.

spondylolisthesis: Forward displacement of a vertebra in relation to the vertebra immediately below.

transverse processes: The ringlike projections on the sides of a vertebra to which muscles and ligaments are attached and, in the chest area, to which the ribs are connected.

vertebroplasty: A minimally invasive procedure to stabilize compressed vertebrae and alleviate pain. A needle is inserted into the compressed portion of a vertebra and surgical cement is injected into it.